Diagnosis and Management of Learning Disabilities

An Interdisciplinary/Lifespan Approach

Diagnosis and Management of Learning Disabilities

An Interdisciplinary/Lifespan Approach

Second Edition

By

Frank R. Brown, III, Ph.D., M.D.
Jeffrey Edwin Gilliam Professor
 of Developmental Disabilities
Medical University of South Carolina
Charleston, South Carolina

Elizabeth H. Aylward, Ph.D.
Assistant Professor
Department of Psychiatry and Behavioral Sciences
The Johns Hopkins University School of Medicine
Baltimore, Maryland

Barbara K. Keogh, Ph.D.
Professor
Department of Education
The University of California, Los Angeles
Los Angeles, California

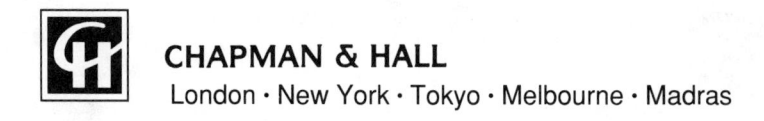

CHAPMAN & HALL
London · New York · Tokyo · Melbourne · Madras

Published by Chapman & Hall, 2–6 Boundary Row, London SE1 8HN

Chapman & Hall, 2–6 Boundary Row, London SE1 8HN, UK

Chapman & Hall, 29 West 35th Street, New York NY 10001, USA

Chapman & Hall Japan, Thomson Publishing Japan, Hirakawacho Nemoto Building, 6F, 1-7-11 Hirakawa-cho, Chiyoda-ku, Tokyo 102, Japan

Chapman & Hall Australia, Thomas Nelson Australia, 102 Dodds Street, South Melbourne, Victoria 3205, Australia

Chapman & Hall India, R. Seshadri, 32 Second Main Road, CIT East, Madras 600,035, India

First edition 1992

©1992 Singular Publishing Group, Inc.

This edition not for sale in North America and Australia; orders from these regions should be referred to Singular Publishing Group, Inc., 4284 41st Street, San Diego, CA 92105, USA.

Typeset in 10/12 Times by So Cal Graphics
Printed in the USA by McNaughton & Gunn

ISBN 0 412 44620 0

Apart from any fair dealing for the purposes of research or private study, or criticism or review, as permitted under the UK Copyright Designs and Patents Act, 1988, this publication may not be reproduced, stored, or transmitted, in any form or by any means, without the prior permission in writing of the publishers, or in the case of reprographic reproduction only in accordance with the terms of the licences issued by the Copyright Licensing Agency in the UK, or in accordance with the terms of licences issued by the appropriate Reproduction rights Organization outside the UK. Enquiries concerning reproduction outside the terms state here should be sent to the publishers at the London address printed on this page.

The publisher makes no representation, express or implied, with regard to the accuracy of the information contained in this book and cannot accept any legal responsibility or liability for any errors or omissions that may be made.

A Catalogue record for this book is available from the British Library

Library of Congress Cataloging-in-Publication data available

Contents

Contributors   viii

Preface   ix

Chapter 1   **Introduction**   1

Learning Disabilities: What Are They? • Definition of Terms • Prevalence of Learning Disabilities • Etiology of Learning Disabilities • The Interdisciplinary Process in Diagnosis and Treatment • Conclusion

Frank R. Brown, III and Elizabeth H. Aylward

PART I: ESTABLISHING THE DIAGNOSIS

Chapter 2   **Learning Disabilities in Preschool Children**   19

Identifying Learning Disabilities in Preschoolers—A Developmental Framework • Applying a Discrepancy Model to Preschool Identification • Additional Diagnostic Criteria • Conclusion

Barbara K. Keogh

Chapter 3   **Neurodevelopmental Evaluation (The Physician's Diagnostic Role in Learning Disabilities)**   35

Identification of Preschool-Age Children at Risk for Learning Disabilities • Neurodevelopmental History and Examination for the School-Age Child • Conclusion

Frank R. Brown, III

Chapter 4   **Psychological Evaluation**   57

History Taking • Psychological Testing • Conclusion

Elizabeth H. Aylward

Chapter 5   **Educational Evaluation**   83

Differences Between Psychological and Educational Assessments • Educational Assessment • Informal Assessment • Conclusion

Judith Margolis and Barbara K. Keogh

Chapter 6	**Language Evaluation**	**101**

Approaches to Assessment • Rule Systems • Auditory Processes • Conclusion

Doris J. Johnson

Chapter 7	**Occupational Therapy Evaluation**	**111**

Occupational Therapy in the Schools • Performance Areas Addressed in the Occupational Therapy Evaluation • Underlying Factors That Interfere With Performance • Conclusion

Winnie Dunn

Chapter 8	**Interdisciplinary Diagnosis**	**123**

Identifying Significant Discrepancy Between Academic Achievement and Intellectual Abilities • Identifying Preschool-Age Children at Risk for Learning Disabilities • Identifying Strengths and Weaknesses in the Learning Style • Identifying Associated Problems • Conclusion

Elizabeth H. Aylward and Frank R. Brown, III

PART II: PLANNING FOR TREATMENT

Chapter 9	**Planning for Treatment of Learning Disabilities and Associated Primary Handicapping Conditions**	**147**

Individualized Educational Plan (IEP) and the Individualized Family Service Plan (IFSP) • Levels of Service • Educational Approaches to Remediate Learning Disabilities • Approaches to Remediating Primary Handicapping Conditions Associated with Learning Disabilities • Accommodations to Circumvent Learning Disabilities • Conclusion

Elizabeth H. Aylward, Frank R. Brown, III, Winnie Dunn, Linda K. Elksnin, and Nick Elksnin

Chapter 10	**Planning for Treatment of Attention-Deficit Hyperactivity Disorder**	**169**

Planning for Remediation of Attention-Deficit Hyperactivity Disorder • Management of Attention-Deficit Hyperactivity Disorder—Environmental Accommodations • Management of Attention-Deficit Hyperactivity Disorder —Use of Psychotropic Medication • Conclusion

Frank R. Brown, III, and Elizabeth H. Aylward

CONTENTS   vii

Chapter 11 **Planning for Treatment of Secondary**   **181**
Handicapping Conditions
Managing Behavior Problems • Managing Secondary Emotional Disturbance • Conclusion

Elizabeth H. Aylward and Frank R. Brown, III

Chapter 12 **Life After High School—Promoting**   **191**
Effective Transition for the Adolescent
with Learning Disabilities
Secondary Program Models • Legislation Affecting Transition Efforts • Making the Transition from High School to Employment • Roles of Professionals and Families • Making the Transition to College • Conclusion

Nick Elksnin and Linda K. Elksnin

Chapter 13 **The Summary Conference**   **205**
Presentation of the Diagnoses • Presentation of Therapeutic Recommendations • Answering Parents' Questions • Planning for Follow-up • Conclusion

Frank R. Brown, III and Elizabeth H. Aylward

GLOSSARY, APPENDICES, REFERENCES,
AND REFERENCE LIST OF TESTS

Glossary   **217**

Appendix A   Parent Interview Form   **221**

Appendix B   Transition Resource List   **224**

References   **226**

Reference List of Tests   **234**

Subject Index   **239**

Contributors

Winnie Dunn, Ph.D., OTR, FAOTA
Professor and Chair
Occupational Therapy Education
University of Kansas Medical Center
Kansas City, Kansas

Linda K. Elksnin, Ph.D.
Associate Professor
Coordinator of Graduate Special Education Programs
The Citadel
Charleston, South Carolina

Nick Elksnin, Ph.D., NCSP
Assistant Professor
Division of Developmental Disabilities
Medical University of South Carolina
Charleston, South Carolina

Doris J. Johnson, Ph.D.
Professor of Learning Disabilities
Program Chair, Program in Learning Disabilities
Northwestern University
Evanston, Illinois

Judith Margolis, Ph.D.
Professor of Education
Department of Special Education
California State University, Los Angeles
Los Angeles, California

PREFACE

Of all childhood disorders, learning disabilities and its concomitant condition, attention-deficit hyperactivity disorder, are by far the most prevalent, occurring in approximately 10 to 15 percent of school-age children. It is important, therefore, that all professionals who work with children understand basic concepts in the identification and treatment of these disorders. Although the second edition of this book, like its predecessor, is written at a level that can be understood by parents or professionals who have little familiarity with learning disorders, it is designed primarily for practitioners who are involved to some degree with diagnosis and treatment of children with learning disabilities.

Children with learning disabilities often have a multitude of problems that span many facets of their lives, including academic, social, emotional, behavioral, and familial. It is imperative, therefore, to consider the total child from several points of view. Practitioners must consider the difficulties encountered in each sphere, as well as the *interactions* among the various problem areas. In the case of the child with learning disabilities, the whole is greater than the sum of the parts.

As stated in the first edition, we believe that an *interdisciplinary* approach allows for the most thorough understanding of the child's problems and needs. When an interdisciplinary approach is used, professionals from many disciplines come together to plan the evaluation, to share results of the assessments they have conducted individually, to discuss how results from evaluation in one discipline relate to results from another discipline, to formulate diagnoses, to plan for treatment and follow-up.

In this second edition, we again have as a primary focus a desire to facilitate an interdisciplinary approach to the diagnosis and treatment of learning disabilities. As a developmental pediatrician, developmental psychologist, and educational psychologist, we endeavor to convey in a simple, straightforward manner what we do when we evaluate and plan treatment for a child with learning disabilities. In this second edition, we wish to emphasize that many of the problems for children with learning disabilities represent chronic handicapping conditions that have an impact across the lifespan of the affected individual. To underscore the need for a lifespan approach to learning disabilities, we introduce two new topics: early (preschool) identification of learning disabilities and promotion of effective transition for the adolescent with learning disabilities. We have asked colleagues in the areas of early identification of learning disabilities, language-based learning disabilities, occupational therapy, and transition programming to help us delineate an interdisciplinary and lifespan approach. We discuss what types of treatments are available for various aspects of the disorder and try to assess objectively the effectiveness of these intervention techniques. Finally, we discuss ways to convey information to parents and to plan for follow-up.

As in the first edition, we have tried intentionally to be brief and direct. Our plan in writing this book was to answer the question "What do you, as a practitioner, do from the moment you first suspect that a child might have a learning disability?" We intend for this book to become a part of the practitioner's working library, as a guide to be used on a day-to-day basis.

CHAPTER 1

Introduction

Frank R. Brown, III
Elizabeth H. Aylward

LEARNING DISABILITIES: WHAT ARE THEY?

Since the term *learning disabilities* was first used by Samuel Kirk in 1962, there has been a great deal of confusion and controversy regarding the nature of this disorder. Special educators, other school personnel, psychologists, physicians, and researchers have proposed many definitions and descriptions of the disorder, a myriad of terms used interchangeably with *learning disabilities*, many theories regarding the etiology of the disorder, and many programs for its remediation.

In 1975 the United States Congress recognized learning disabilities as a handicapping condition and assured free and appropriate education for all children with learning disabilities. At this time, it became imperative that schools devise a system for making decisions about the eligibility of individual students for participation in the required special education programs. The federal government's definition of *specific learning disabilities* was included in the Education for All Handicapped Children Act as part of Public Law 94-142 (1975). The definition cited in the act is as follows:

> Specific learning disability means a disorder in one or more of the basic psychological processes involved in the understanding or in using language, spoken or written, which may manifest itself in an imperfect ability to listen, think, speak, read, write, spell, or to do

mathematical calculations. The term includes such conditions as perceptual handicaps, brain injury, minimal brain dysfunction, dyslexia, and developmental aphasia. The term does not apply to children who have learning problems which are primarily the result of visual, hearing, or motor handicaps, of mental retardation, or emotional disturbance, or of environmental, cultural or economic disadvantages. (Public Law 94-142, 34 C.F.R. 300.5 [b] [9])

To further clarify the term *learning disabilities*, the government provided educators with a separate set of federal regulations for the implementation of Public Law 94-142. These regulations are the "Procedures for Evaluation of Specific Learning Disabilities" (U.S. Office of Education, 1977). According to these regulations, a child has a specific learning disability if:

1. The child does not achieve commensurate with his or her age and ability levels in one or more of seven specific areas when provided with learning experiences appropriate for the child's age and ability level.
2. The team finds that a child has a severe discrepancy between achievement and intellectual ability in one or more of the following areas:
   a. oral expression
   b. listening comprehension
   c. written expression
   d. basic reading skills
   e. reading comprehension
   f. mathematics calculation
   g. mathematics reasoning. (p. 65083)

Despite federal efforts to clarify the definition of learning disabilities, many professionals launched criticisms based on the definition's ambiguity, redundancy, and unnecessary restrictions (see Berk, 1984, for further discussion). To address these criticisms, the National Joint Committee for Learning Disabilities (NJCLD) (1981), composed of representatives from six professional organizations, proposed a new definition, which was presented as follows:

Learning disabilities is a generic term that refers to a heterogeneous group of disorders manifested by significant difficulties in the acquisition and use of listening, speaking, reading, writing, reasoning, or mathematical abilities. These disorders are intrinsic to the individual and presumed to be due to central nervous system dysfunction.

INTRODUCTION

> Even though learning disabilities may occur concomitantly with other handicapping conditions (e.g., sensory impairment, mental retardation, social and emotional disturbance) or environmental influences (e.g., cultural differences, insufficient/inappropriate instruction, psychogenic factors), it is not the direct result of those conditions or influences. (p. 5).

Most school systems have used a combination of these definitions and regulations as the basis for establishing procedures to identify children with learning disabilities. In doing so, the attempt has been made to determine the existence of "severe discrepancy" between achievement and intellectual ability in the individual. Because no federal guidelines have been established for defining "severe discrepancy," state and local education agencies have been forced to establish their own procedures for measuring achievement and intellectual ability, and for identifying "severe discrepancy." Even within states or regions where procedures have been established, many different approaches are used by various professionals to identify students with learning disabilities. Especially for parents and professionals not specializing in the identification of learning disabilities on a day-to-day basis, there continues to be a great deal of confusion in determining whether any particular child is or is not learning disabled.

When eligibility definitions for learning disabilities were developed in response to Public Law 94-142, there was little initial focus on infants and toddlers at risk for subsequent learning disabilities, and eligibility definitions for learning disabilities were developed solely with school-age children in mind. In 1986, Public Law 99-457 was introduced, focusing on development of comprehensive, coordinated, multidisciplinary, and interagency programs of early intervention services for infants and toddlers who were handicapped and their families. As a result of this legislation, there has evolved a thrust to identify preschool-age children "at risk" for subsequent developmental disabilities, including learning disabilities. Professionals involved with preschoolers at risk for learning disabilities have been forced to develop alternatives to discrepancy definitions of this disorder. Some of these alternative approaches will be discussed in subsequent chapters.

Focus has expanded to include not only preschoolers at risk for learning disabilities, but also young adults with ongoing learning disabilities. In 1984, the Carl D. Perkins Vocational Act (P. L. 98-524) mandated services to aid in the transition from high school to post-high school for individuals with learning disabilities. As a result, professionals are now accountable to individuals with learning disabilities across the life span of their disability.

DEFINITION OF TERMS

It is our opinion that much of the confusion regarding learning disabilities reflects a lack of understanding of the underlying basis and natural history of this disorder. This lack of understanding is reflected in the large number of terms that often are used imprecisely and inappropriately to suggest more understanding of the disorder than is justified. These include terms such as *specific learning disability, minimal brain dysfunction, attention-deficit hyperactivity disorder,* and *dyslexia.* In this book the use of terms reflects our philosophy regarding the neurological basis of learning disabilities. These definitions are presented in a format that, it is hoped, will clarify a distinction that the authors wish to make between primary (neurologically based) and secondary (derivative of primary) disorders.

Primary (Neurologically Based) Handicapping Conditions

The primary handicapping conditions for children with learning disabilities are assumed to reflect brain "damage," albeit often of subtle degree and undetectable given current medical technologies. Like all disorders, mild degrees of brain damage are far more common than more serious degrees. This is reflected in the high incidence of learning disabilities and associated primary handicapping conditions, in comparison to more serious neurological dysfunctions, such as mental retardation and cerebral palsy.

The brain damage assumed in children with learning disabilities is typically diffuse, meaning that multiple brain functions are affected. Two important areas of neurological functioning for the child with learning disabilities are cognitive and motor skills. Diffuse cognitive dysfunction might involve expressive or receptive language, visual-spatial perceptual abilities, or the ability to focus and maintain attention. Diffuse motor dysfunction might include weaknesses in gross motor, fine motor, or oral motor skills.

The typical child with learning disabilities will show some mixture of difficulties in cognitive and motor function. Because the motor and cognitive difficulties frequently are subtle, parents and professionals sometimes may not appreciate their impact on the child. It is especially important to look not just at the "tip of the iceberg" (i.e., see the obvious and most major handicapping condition), but also to be alert to less obvious associated difficulties.

The primary handicapping conditions most often seen in children with learning disabilities (and requiring careful definition) are defined as follows.

Learning Disabilities

In the case of the school-age child, the definition of learning disabilities that we use is based on the 1975 federal definition included as part of Public Law 94-142, the 1977 U.S. Office of Education (U.S.O.E.) regulations, and the 1981 NJCLD definitions. We limit the use of the term *learning disability* in the school-age child to a condition whereby an individual's academic achievement level is significantly below the level that would be predicted from the level of intellectual ability. The cause for the discrepancy between academic achievement and intellectual ability is presumed to be neurologically based. Although learning disabilities can occur concomitantly with other handicapping conditions or environmental influences, they are not the direct result of these conditions or influences. Learning disabilities can occur in the areas of listening, speaking, reading, writing, reasoning, or mathematical abilities. Primary focus, however, is placed on learning disabilities in three areas:

READING. A specific learning disability in reading (also termed *dyslexia*) occurs when individual reading skills (e.g., word attack, reading comprehension) or general reading ability are significantly below the level that would be predicted from the individual's level of intellectual ability, assuming other handicapping conditions or environmental influences have been ruled out. If the reading disability is thought to be caused by an overall weakness in language skills, it may be referred to as a "language-based" learning disability.

MATHEMATICS. A specific learning disability in mathematics (also termed *dyscalculia*) occurs when individual math skills (e.g., acquisition of number facts, written calculations, mathematical reasoning) or general mathematical ability are significantly below the level that would be predicted from the individual's level of intellectual ability, assuming other handicapping conditions or environmental influences have been ruled out.

WRITTEN LANGUAGE. A specific learning disability in written language (also termed *dysgraphia*) occurs when individual written language skills (e.g., spelling, application of grammar, punctuation, usage skills, organization of thoughts in writing) or general written language ability are significantly below the level that would be predicted from the individual's level of intellectual ability, assuming other handicapping conditions or environmental influences have been ruled out. Although it may be considered a specific learning disability in itself, poor handwriting is not included in the term *dysgraphia*, as we use it.

In response to P. L. 99-457 and the desire to identify children with learning disabilities as early as possible, many professionals have attempted to identify preschoolers "at risk" for subsequent learning disabilities. We feel, as discussed in Chapter 8, that there currently is no diagnostic procedure(s) that reliably identifies the preschool child who subsequently will demonstrate significant discrepancies between cognitive functioning and academic achievement (i.e., will evidence learning disabilities). There are, however, many identifiable factors that predict subsequent *slow academic achievement*, if not necessarily academic achievement that is deviant from cognitive expectation. Children who are at risk for subsequent *slow academic achievement* (not necessarily learning disabilities) may be identified by delays in language, visual-perception, attention span and/or impulse control, and problems with behavior. For the remainder of the book, we will use the term "at risk for learning difficulties" to refer to those children who can be expected to encounter difficulties in academic achievement, whether or not these difficulties represent true learning disabilities.

Attention-Deficit Hyperactivity Disorder (ADHD)

The definition used by the authors is based on the criteria set in the *Diagnostic and Statistical Manual of Mental Disorders (Third Edition-Revised)* of the American Psychiatric Association (1987). To be diagnosed as having attention-deficit hyperactivity disorder, a child must meet criteria for developmentally inappropriate degrees of inattention (e.g., failure to finish things he or she starts, failure to listen, easy distractibility, difficulty in concentrating or sticking to a play activity), criteria for impulsivity (e.g., acting before thinking, shifting from one activity to another, difficulty in organization, need for supervision, frequent calling out in class, and difficulty awaiting turns), and exhibit hyperactivity (e.g., run or climb excessively, have difficulty sitting still or staying seated).

We attempt to distinguish between a child with a developmentally inappropriate inattention and poor impulse control, and a child who simply exhibits an exaggerated motor activity level. In essence we are saying clinically that children may exhibit attention deficit disorder with or without hyperactivity. This distinction and separation of the issues of attention deficit disorder and hyperactivity was indicated more clearly in the earlier version of the *Diagnostic and Statistical Manual-III* (American Psychiatric Association, 1980), in that attention deficit disorder was described as occurring in the presence or absence of hyperactivity. The separation of these issues is somewhat obscured in the current term attention-deficit hyperactivity disorder, which tends to imply that deficits of attention span and impulse control will occur in accompaniment with excessive motor activity (hyperactivity). Despite reservations about amalgamating these clinical entities, we will adhere throughout the text to the newer terminology of attention-deficit hyperactivity disorder (ADHD). It is important additionally to realize that many children have attention-deficit hyperactivity disorder without learning disabilities, and many children with learning disabilities do not have attention-deficit hyperactivity disorder. The two disorders are, however, often seen concomitantly.

Minimal Brain Dysfunction (MBD)

We use this term to refer to the child who has a mixture of some or all of the subtle cognitive and motor dysfunctions described previously. Components of MBD may include learning disabilities, language disabilities, other inconsistencies among various cognitive functions, ADHD, gross-, fine-, and oral-motor dyscoordinations. What is clear from this listing is that ADHD is part of a larger syndrome that originally was termed MBD. Developmentalists and educators have, with the term ADHD, focused on that part of this larger MBD syndrome that they felt was most significant in terms of school dysfunction, that is, deficits of attention span and impulse control. Clearly, there are a number of children who exhibit a much wider spectrum of symptoms than are accounted for by the term ADHD, and for these children the term MBD may still be an appropriate description.

Secondary (Derivative of Primary) Handicapping Conditions

Unlike the primary handicapping conditions described previously, secondary handicapping conditions do not have a direct neurological basis. They are instead the *result* of the primary handicapping conditions, especially when the primary handicapping conditions have not been managed properly. The most common secondary handicapping conditions are poor self-concept and inappropriate attention-seeking behaviors. Poor self-concept is often the result of academic failure, especially when the child is blamed or told that the failure is due to lack of motivation. When children with learning disabilities are unable to receive recognition for positive achievements (e.g., academic success) they sometimes resort to inappropriate behaviors to obtain recognition, despite the fact that the recognition often is negative. In addition to these two common secondary handicapping conditions, children with learning disabilities also may exhibit such secondary characteristics as poor peer relationships, compliance problems, oppositional behaviors, depression, school phobia, and other problems of adjustment.

Slow Learner

Although children with learning disabilities demonstrate slow achievement in some or all academic areas, their cognitive functioning usually is average or better. The authors wish to distinguish between children with learning disabilities and children labeled "slow learners." *Slow learner* is a term used to describe the child whose learning ability in all areas is delayed in comparison to children of the same chronological age. These children are characterized by low-normal to borderline intelligence, with corresponding slow academic progress. These children are not considered learning disabled because there is no discrepancy between cognitive expectations and academic achievement. Although generally not eligible for special education services, these children often are in need of a modified curriculum and more individual attention than their nonaffected peers. The authors will not address this population except to point out that the number of slow learners is at least as great as the number of students with learning disabilities, and to express an opinion that these students need and deserve special education services as much as students with learning disabilities.

PREVALENCE OF LEARNING DISABILITIES

Failure to define terms precisely has led to confusion over prevalence rates. Prevalence rates for learning disabilities range between 3% and 15% of the school-age population and vary according to geographic area (Sixth Annual Report to Congress, 1984). Boys are diagnosed as being learning disabled four to eight times as often as girls (Marsh, Gearhart, & Gearhart, 1978). Although there are no definite figures regarding the prevalence of ADHD within the population with learning disabilities, estimates vary from 33% to 80% (Interagency Committee on Learning Disabilities, 1987). Safer and Allen (1976) estimated that approximately 30% of hyperactive children are learning disabled, although recent work by Halpern, Gittleman, and Klein (1984) puts the figure at 10%.

ETIOLOGY OF LEARNING DISABILITIES

In discussing learning disabilities, many parents ask, "Why is my child learning disabled?" In most cases, professionals must answer, "I don't know," because the etiology of learning disabilities rarely can be determined for certain. However, it is known that the incidence of learning disabilities is increased among family members of children with the disorder, suggesting a genetic link. Parents (especially fathers) sometimes will remark that their child's difficulties are similar to problems they experienced as children. Children who have experienced certain types of birth trauma (e.g., lack of sufficient oxygen at or around the time of birth, difficult delivery, prematurity) also have a higher incidence of learning disabilities, as well as other developmental delays. However, it must be kept in mind that causality cannot be presumed from the fact that two conditions frequently occur together. It is, therefore, rarely possible to pinpoint for certain the exact "cause" of the problem in an individual child.

As the term *learning disabilities* usually is defined, the assumption is made that the disorder is due, at least in part, to some type of neurological irregularity. The nature of the irregularity has, however, been much debated. One general view presumes that the neurological abnormalities are a consequence of aberrant organization or dysfunction of the central nervous system (Critchley, 1970; Hinshelwood, 1917; and others). The neurological "deficits" referred to in this "deficit" model are very subtle and cannot be recognized or localized using present technologies. An alternative view is the "no defect" or maturational lag hypothesis (Bender, 1957; Kinsbourne, 1975; and others). This hypothesis suggests that children with learning disabilities merely possess a slower rate of normal development of neural processes relevant to the acquisition of academic skills. It implies that children with learning disabilities eventually will develop the requisite neural processes and then will learn with normal or near-normal facility (McKeever & VanDeventer, 1975).

Witelson (1977) points out that there is no empirical support for the hypothesis implied by the "developmental lag" model that children with learning disabilities eventually "catch up" and become normal. We agree that most children with learning disabilities, especially those with a concomitant ADHD, continue to demonstrate weaknesses in academic achievement, despite all remedial efforts, well into adolescence and beyond. As Witelson (1977) notes, a "deficit model" does not preclude the manifestation of a lag in development of cognitive skills. Most disorders, she states, result in test performance that is at least superficially comparable to that of normal children at some earlier chronological age.

Parents will occasionally ask if their child is learning disabled or merely suffering from some type of developmental lag or delay. The authors generally would answer these parents by agreeing that the child does, indeed, have a delay that makes him or her appear "immature" or poorly developed in certain areas. Parents would, however, be discouraged from believing that the child will "catch up" (with or without intervention) and eventually appear normal. Of course, children with mild delays, especially if they are bright, may learn ways to circumvent their weaknesses. However, it would be a mistake to say that the neurological abnormalities underlying these weaknesses do not continue to exist. It also should be noted that individuals with learning disabilities often experience few difficulties once they have finished school because they can avoid situations that demand those skills that caused problems for them in the school setting.

It may be inappropriate to assume that all symptomatology related to learning disabilities and especially ADHD, necessarily will prove ultimately to be so maladaptive. Levine, Brooks, and Shonkoff (1980) have suggested that many of the symptoms of ADHD may have some positive facets and potential for good prognosis. The child with disabling distractibility in school may prove to make interesting observations with less confined associations as an adult. The child with ADHD and fast paced cognitive tempo may prove to be an extremely productive adult. In essence, when the child with ADHD is permitted as an adult to develop his or her own strengths (and opportunity to bypass areas of weakness), the "disorder" of attention-deficit hyperactivity disorder may evolve into some areas of strength.

Finally, in discussing the etiology of learning disabilities, it must be mentioned that investigators over the years have proposed many theories to explain what is "wrong" in the brains of children with learning disabilities. For example, it has been proposed that these children suffer from inadequate lateralization of the brain hemispheres, from language processing deficits, from deficits in visual discrimination, from poor auditory-visual integration, from poor visual closure, or from poor auditory sequential memory. (See Johnson, 1981, for a thorough history of these theories.) We will not add to this list of theories by attempting to identify *the* underlying problem that leads to learning disabilities. We assume, however, that children with learning disabilities are not a homogeneous group. Learning disabilities are not the result of one etiology (e.g., genetics or birth trauma) and are not caused by one type of deficit (e.g., language-processing or lack of cerebral lateralization). The diagnostic process is primarily designed to identify which children actually are experiencing learning disabilities, not to theorize about possible underlying causes.

THE INTERDISCIPLINARY PROCESS IN DIAGNOSIS AND TREATMENT

What is the Interdisciplinary Process?

We wish to distinguish between a *multidisciplinary* and an *interdisciplinary* process. The former involves a series of individual evaluations and treatment plans by several disciplines (e.g., special education, medicine, psychology). The latter involves a comprehensive integrated and systematic approach, whereby professionals from several disciplines come together to plan the diagnostic procedures to be used, carry out a variety of evaluative procedures, meet again to share the results of the evaluations, formulate diagnoses based on these evaluations, work together to devise appropriate treatment procedures, and assign responsibility to individual team members for carrying out various parts of the plan.

Who Is Involved?

The interdisciplinary process can be carried out in a variety of settings. One common setting would be a diagnostic and evaluation clinic, whose staff probably would include physicians, psychologists, and special educators, as well as professionals in allied fields such as speech-language therapy and occupational and physical therapy. In this case, outside professionals who are familiar with the child, especially school personnel, would be asked to participate. Alternatively, the interdisciplinary process could be initiated by the school, with participation solicited from the child's physician and any other outside professionals familiar with the child. An individual professional working privately with the child, such as a physician, private language therapist, tutor, or psychologist, might initiate and coordinate the process. On rare occasions, the procedure might even be initiated by parents, who would make arrangements for all of the professionals working with their child to meet for interdisciplinary diagnosis and development of therapeutic recommendations.

Regardless of the setting, the interdisciplinary process minimally should consist of a physician, psychologist, and educator. Other professionals who may be beneficial in the process would include any other school personnel familiar with the child (school principal, special education teacher, school psychologist, school nurse, speech-language therapist, occupational or physical therapist, guidance counselor, social worker, regular classroom teachers), as well as nonschool personnel (physician, psychologists who may have been enlisted independently by the family for evaluation, therapists, social workers from outside agencies, nursery school teachers, community health nurses, and private tutors).

Nonschool professionals must, of course, respect the fact that the school, as the primary service provider, has regulations and procedures that must be followed. These professionals should assist school personnel in determining whether the child meets criteria for diagnosis of learning disabilities by providing information about the child to which the school may not have immediate access (assuming, of course, that the child's parents have agreed to such disclosure). They should assist in the development of appropriate in-school interventions, again by providing additional information about the child that may be relevant in deciding which strategies will be most effective. Nonschool professionals can play a major role in devising out-of-school interventions that may augment the program provided by the school (e.g., instructing parents in behavior management strategies, providing extracurricular activities that might build the child's self-concept, or suggesting counseling for parents whose expectations are unrealistic). Of course, the physician is a vital member of the team when decisions are being made regarding the need for medication to control ADHD.

Certain nonschool professionals, especially the child's physician, may be in an excellent position to ensure continuity of appropriate services, even if the child moves from school to school. Because most children have regular contact with their physician and because parents usually are willing to share information freely with the physician, he or she can monitor the child's treatment and progress. Children who might otherwise "fall through the cracks" of the educational system can be assured appropriate ongoing services.

Finally, nonschool personnel should, when necessary, monitor the school's approach to diagnosis and treatment. Unfortunately, some schools still are using outdated methods for identifying children with learning disabilities. Nonschool personnel may need to make certain that the children they represent are not disqualified from service because they do not meet certain inappropriate criteria (e.g., large subtest scatter on the intelligence test). Nonschool personnel may need to monitor the type and amount of special education service the school is planning to provide. For example, if a child needs speech therapy but the school does not employ a speech therapist, the school may not be willing to include the therapy as part of the treatment plan. Nonschool personnel may need to intervene on behalf of the child.

Of course, the primary goal of the interdisciplinary team is to serve the child. Team members, both school and nonschool personnel, should view the interdisciplinary process as an opportunity to educate one another regarding their individual disciplines, as well as an opportunity to provide optimal service to the child and family.

How Does the Interdisciplinary Process Work?

The first step in the interdisciplinary process is generally some type of *prescreening*. This step may be done by the case manager or by a committee and involves determining whether the child is experiencing difficulty that warrants thorough evaluation. This determination generally is made by talking with the person who initiated the referral (e.g., parents, teacher, physician) to obtain a description of the nature and history of the problems the child is experiencing. When possible, it is beneficial for those conducting the prescreening process to review records or talk briefly with individuals other than the referral source.

The most important aspect of the prescreening process is to determine what types of evaluation are most appropriate and will lead to the most fruitful results. Just as a physician determines what types of lab tests to conduct on the basis of the patient's symptoms, the individual(s) conducting the prescreening must determine from a description of the child's problems whether it would be more productive to explore the possibility of learning disabilities rather than other disorders (e.g., serious emotional disturbance). More specifically, the prescreening process will allow the case manager to make arrangements, when necessary, for evaluations from allied professionals (e.g., speech and language therapist, occupational therapist, physical therapist).

Finally, the individual(s) conducting the prescreening process should determine whether any evaluations have already been conducted that will be relevant in the formulation of the diagnoses and therapeutic recommendations. Although it is not necessary that the case manager determine precisely what evaluations will be carried out before the diagnostic process is initiated, some preplanning may reduce the number of visits the family must make to the clinic, reduce redundancy among the evaluations, and ensure that the concerns of the referring party are addressed thoroughly.

After the prescreening team or case manager has determined which evaluations will be most productive, individual professionals conduct the appropriate evaluations. These evaluations generally consist of a thorough history (obtained through review of records and interviews with the parents, teachers, and child), as well as assessment with specific tests. The types of evaluation procedures employed by the physician, psychologist, educator, and allied professionals are described thoroughly in Chapters 3 through 7. Some of the options currently available to identify preschool-age children "at risk" for subsequent learning difficulties are discussed in Chapter 2.

After the individual professionals have conducted their evaluations, a case conference is held during which each professional shares the results of his or her evaluation. By reviewing Chapters 2 through 7, individual team members will have the necessary background to understand the evaluation techniques employed by each of the various disciplines. It is important, for example, for the special educator to understand how the physician arrived at a diagnosis of ADHD. It is equally important for the physician to understand the nature of the tests used by the psychologist to determine the level of the child's cognitive abilities. By understanding each discipline's evaluative procedures, team members can better understand the data presented and its relationship to their own data, suggest alternative interpretations to the data, monitor the appropriateness of the evaluation procedures for individual children, and identify areas in which information is incomplete.

After the data have been presented, the case manager will need to summarize the data presented and formulate tentative diagnoses to be discussed by the team. (Chapter 8 describes how the information gathered by each of the team members can be integrated to arrive at appropriate diagnoses.) Following discussion of the data presented, team members should be able to agree on a list of the primary and secondary handicapping conditions that are interfering with successful performance. On occasion, however, team members may decide that further evaluation is necessary before the diagnoses can be formulated. In this case, final diagnoses are postponed until a later meeting.

After diagnoses have been established, the interdisciplinary team should formulate a general treatment plan. For example, it might be determined that the child should receive special education services in mathematics and written language, that a trial on medication for ADHD should be initiated, and that the parents should be provided with some training in behavior management strategies. Just as individual team members need to understand the evaluation procedures employed by professionals from other disciplines, it is important that they understand the various treatment strategies used. The special education teacher, for example, needs to understand what should be expected from a child treated with medication for ADHD. Similarly, the psychologist needs to understand what types of reading programs are used by special educators to deal with a child who demonstrates language processing difficulties. By understanding the various treatment modalities available to the child, team members can better determine which treatments should be used, when and how they should be employed (e.g., all treatments started simultaneously or various treatments added in increments), how to evaluate their effectiveness, and how to determine when they are no longer needed. Strategies for treatment of primary and secondary handicapping conditions are discussed in Chapters 9, 10, and 11.

Because we acknowledge the chronic nature of learning disabilities, as well as the importance of integrating the young adult with learning disabilities into the community, strategies for effective transition are discussed in Chapter 12.

The team should not attempt at the time of the initial interdisciplinary conference to develop specific goals and objectives, timelines for accomplishing their aims, or criteria for success. Instead, individual team members should be assigned responsibility for ensuring that the general areas of the treatment plan are refined further and implemented. The team should determine, however, what procedures will be used to coordinate and monitor the implementation of the general treatment plan. Procedures for follow-up and reevaluation also should be addressed.

Following this interdisciplinary case conference, the case manager (or other person appointed by the team) will be responsible for sharing the results of the evaluation, the diagnostic formulation, and the general therapeutic recommendations with the parents. Strategies for parent counseling are discussed in Chapter 13. This step is necessary to promote the parents' understanding and acceptance of their child's disorders and to elicit their cooperation in treatment. Parents of the school-age child with learning disabilities often are encouraged to participate in the development of the Individualized Educational Plan (IEP) at the child's school (Chapter 9). With the introduction of P. L. 99-457, Individualized Family Service Plans (IFSPs) are required for outlining appropriate services for at-risk children and their families. Parents' contribution to the development of these plans will be enhanced greatly if they have been previously presented with information regarding their child's disorders, been given the opportunity to ask the questions necessary to clarify their understanding of the situation, and had a chance to discuss treatment options.

CONCLUSION

The field of learning disabilities has matured tremendously since the term was introduced in 1962. However, there is still a great deal of confusion and misunderstanding, even among professionals who diagnose and treat children with learning disabilities on a regular basis. Part of the reason for misunderstanding involves the interdisciplinary nature of the disorder. Because the child with learning disabilities often exhibits problems that generally are treated by professionals in different disciplines, it has been difficult for individual professionals to deal effectively with the total child. For this reason, an interdisciplinary approach is vitally important. By understanding better the diagnostic and treatment tools available to each discipline involved with the child, individual professionals can work together more effectively for the *total* well-being of the child and family.

PART 1

ESTABLISHING THE DIAGNOSIS

CHAPTER 2

Learning Disabilities in Preschool Children

Barbara K. Keogh

Interest in learning disabilities in young children stems in part from the recognition that development is malleable in the early years, that appropriate services may alleviate or at least moderate the severity of problems, and that secondary, compounding problems may be prevented. Accumulating findings from numerous studies document real, and sometimes dramatic, gains in young children's cognitive and educational competencies as a result of early intervention. The Perry Preschool Project, for example, is a longitudinal study carried out over 20 years. Compared to control peers, in adolescence the children who received early intervention had fewer subsequent special educational needs, fewer delinquencies, and in general were educationally and personally more competent (Berruta-Clement, Schweinhart, Barnett, Epstein, & Weikart, 1984).

These findings are consistent with many clinical reports of early diagnosis and intervention and with findings from the eleven projects providing early intervention with children who are disadvantaged reviewed by Lazar and Darlington (1982). A meta-analysis of 74 early intervention studies with preschoolers who were handicapped also documented positive effects when the outcome measures were IQ, social competence, language, motor development, and pre-academic skills (Casto & Mastropieri, 1986). Based on a review of relevant studies, Mastropieri (1988) concluded that early intervention does produce strong effects with a variety of preschool children who are handicapped or at risk, that deficits in specific components of reading may be identified and trained, and that there are reliable measures for determining an achievement-aptitude discrepancy in young children. Taken as a whole, the findings to date argue for the importance of early recognition and intervention with young children with learning disabilities.

The focus on the early years has resulted in a proliferating research literature and in changes in policy and legislation which allow, and in some cases, guarantee services to preschoolers with learning disabilities and their families. Following the lead in P. L. 94-142 (1975), the Education for All Handicapped Children Act, both P. L. 99-457 (1986), the Education of the Handicapped Amendments, and the Human Services Reauthorization Act of 1986 acknowledge learning disabilities in young children as a handicapping condition. These acts call for early identification and for programs of treatment or intervention which include both children and their families. Indeed, the focus for preschoolers deemed to be at risk for learning disabilities has shifted from the individual child and an Individualized Educational Plan (IEP) to families and an Individualized Family Services Plan (IFSP).

The goals specified in the legislation are necessary and worthwhile. Our challenge is to find methods and techniques to implement the mandates, because there are a number of ambiguities and unanswered questions about learning disabilities in young children. Two related questions of importance are: How are learning disabilities expressed in young children? How do we identify learning disabilities in the preschool years? The answers to these questions require us to consider learning disabilities within a developmental framework; that is, to consider learning disabilities against a backdrop of expected developmental patterns and accomplishments.

IDENTIFYING LEARNING DISABILITIES IN PRESCHOOLERS— A DEVELOPMENTAL FRAMEWORK

There are many rich descriptions of characteristics of "typical" children at different ages, and these descriptions provide broad, normative expectancies. A number of tests and surveys document behaviors and skills expected of children at given ages. Well-known and widely used approaches include the Gesell Developmental Schedules (Gesell & Amatruda, 1947), the Bayley Scales of Infant Development (Bayley, 1969), and the Minnesota Child Development Inventory (Ireton & Thwing, 1974) They provide ways to describe systematically the developmental status of children at particular time points. It is important to remember, however, that within each age period there is a wide range of individual differences and many different patterns of growth. A visit to any preschool illustrates dramatically the variations among preschoolers in physical size and motor skills, in language facility, and in social competencies. Some children will be "typical" in most developmental areas, others will be accelerated or delayed in all, and still others will have uneven patterns of skills. Important considerations from a developmental perspective involve the significance of these differences as predictors of subsequent developmental problems, and their stability and continuity over time.

These points become particularly important when we attempt to identify learning disabilities early on, as it is not entirely clear which characteristics or "signs" are necessary for confident identification or diagnosis. There also is uncertainty about the long term significance of many early indicators. Placing learning disabilities in the preschool years within a developmental framework allows us to consider a broad range of characteristics, including pre-academic accomplishments. It also underscores the need to consider a given child's attributes and problems against a backdrop of normal developmental expectancies, as a particular sign or behavior may be age-specific rather than problem-specific. Inability to follow a sequence of verbal instructions is not unusual in 2-year-olds, but is surprising in 5-year-olds; copying complex geometric designs is too difficult a task for 3-year-olds but is successfully mastered by most kindergartners. The point to be emphasized is that understanding the significance of particular signs or symptoms in the diagnosis of learning disabilities assumes a developmental framework.

How we define learning disabilities and the techniques we use for assessment have important practical implications for services for children and their families. This approach is especially true as definitions and assessments lead to clinical and educational decisions about who is identified, who receives services, and what kinds of services are provided. More important, the questions force us to consider what we mean by learning disabilities in the early childhood years. Paraphrasing the definition in P. L. 94-142, specific learning disabilities in older children and adults describe problems in basic psychological processes or language which impair or affect abilities in higher order literacy and mathematical skills. This component of the definition has led to an emphasis on the expression of learning disabilities in school-age children. It also has led to an emphasis on learning disabilities defined as a discrepancy between actual and expected achievement in school subjects (e.g., reading, arithmetic, spelling). The discrepancy definition has itself been challenged, but is still widely accepted as an important criterion of learning disabilities.

An interesting practical problem arises when we attempt to use a discrepancy definition to identify learning disabilities in children who have not reached school age. Three- and 4-year-old children are not expected to have basic reading or mathematic calculation skills, nor to have well-developed abilities in written expression, reading comprehension, or mathematics reasoning, all components of the federal guidelines for identification. Thus, it is difficult to apply a discrepancy definition using these educational accomplishments or outcomes. Limiting learning disabilities to an educational frame of reference almost precludes identification in the early years. Because of this situation, a *neurodevelopmental* perspective is important.

McCarthy (1989) suggests that the federal definition of learning disabilities found in P. L. 94-142 should be modified for young children so that a severe discrepancy is defined in terms of differences between *actual* developmental accomplishments and *expected* developmental milestones and/or intellectual ability. She proposes that the achievement domains of importance should be the precursors of academic skills, specifically, oral expression, listening comprehension, prewriting, prereading, and premathematics skills. She also suggests that basic processes or abilities of importance in the preschool years ". . . include, but are not limited to, attention, memory, perceptual and perceptual-motor skills, thinking, language, and nonverbal abilities" (p. 70).

McCarthy's approach is similar to that of the National Joint Committee on Learning Disabilities (Leigh, 1986) which proposes that learning disabilities in the preschool years may be expressed as deficits in areas of language, speech, and reasoning, and may co-occur with problems in social interaction and in motor skills or self-regulation. Implicit in both approaches is the notion that the young child with learning disabilities has abilities and behaviors that are different or discrepant from normative expectancies, and that these differences are not explainable by sensory limitations, general cognitive deficits, or disadvantaged environments. This definitional approach is consistent with the one applied to older children and adults, except that the discrepancy is based on developmental milestones and pre-academic skills rather than on intellectual ability and specific academic accomplishments.

Is a Discrepancy Definition Useful for Preschoolers?

The idea that a learning disability in preschoolers can be recognized through a discrepancy analysis is an appealing one, as most adults have general ideas about what children of a given age "ought" to be like, and therefore recognize deficits or differences from these norms. There are many tests or surveys that describe normative characteristics of children at different developmental stages or periods. Nonetheless, determination of a significant discrepancy is not without problems. Practical concerns relate to which developmental domains or dimensions are important, how they should be measured, and how great a difference must be to warrant consideration as a serious discrepancy. Identifying a specific disability may be particularly difficult in the early years, as language or motor deficits may be indicators of general cognitive delay as well as of a specific learning disability.

There are numerous children, however, who reach expected developmental milestones in most ability areas, but who are markedly slow or behind in the mastery of specific accomplishments. Rather than general cognitive or intellectual delay, these children show signs of specific disabilities. They are similar to school-age children with learning disabilities who have discrepancies between general ability and specific academic accomplishments, except that in young children the discrepancies are between general ability and pre-academic skills. One reasonable approach to identification of preschool children with learning disabilities, then, is to establish a significant discrepancy between general cognitive ability and specific pre-academic skills. To implement the discrepancy model, two practical questions to be considered are: Which pre-academic skills should be assessed? How may they be assessed accurately?

Considering first the question of which pre-academic skills, there is some agreement that certain indicators or deficits in the early years are particularly important signals of possible problems. From a comprehensive review of the literature from education, psychology, medicine, and related fields, the most frequently cited symptoms or indicators in the preschool years were: delays or disturbance in language understanding and usage; deficits in visual perception/visual problem solving; deficits in attention span and/or impulse control; and behavior problems, including oppositional, non-compliant, and avoidant behaviors (Keogh, Major-Kingsley, Omori-Gordon, & Reed, 1982). These problem areas deserve brief discussion as they provide a potentially useful description of young children with learning disabilities.

Language Problems

It should not surprise us that language problems are considered a significant indicator of learning disabilities, given the importance of language in educational and personal-social competencies. Language processing abilities consistently are found to be associated with reading problems, and many different kinds of language impairments have been implicated. These range from generalized delay to specific deficits or disturbances, including problems in receptive vocabulary, syntax, phonemic awareness, and phonological production, all problems that are identifiable in 2- and 3-year-olds. A recent study is illustrative. Scarborough (1990) summarized the early language picture of children who are dyslexic as typically evidencing vocabulary deficiencies, poor rhyming and recitation skills, and phonemic awareness deficits at 3 to 4 years of age; and, as 2-year-olds to have produced shorter and simpler sentences and to have more pronunciation problems than normally developing peers. Other investigators also find that preschool tests of expressive and receptive syntax and semantics are associated with later problems in reading and spelling, and that children with learning disabilities have particular problems with complex language demands such as narratives or story telling. Thus, there is considerable evidence that suggests that language delay or disturbance may be key indicators of potential learning disabilities.

A number of developmental tests include assessment of both receptive and expressive language domains (e.g., the Bayley Scales of Infant Development, Bayley, 1969; the Battelle Developmental Inventory, Newborg, Stock, Wnek, Guidubaldi, & Svinicki, 1984), and there also are language specific measures (e.g., the Sequenced Inventory of Communication Development, Hedrick, Prather, & Tobin, 1975; the Reynell-Zinkin Scales, Reynell, 1979). It should be emphasized, however, that language problems are not necessarily specific to learning disabilities, but also may be indicators of other developmental problems, particularly cognitive delay (see Hecht, 1986, for discussion). It should also be emphasized that there is considerable variation in how and when children achieve early language milestones, and that language delay does not necessarily signal problem development. However, given the importance of language in children's intellectual and social development, serious discrepancies from normative expectancies deserve attention as signs of possible learning disabilities.

Attention-Deficit Hyperactivity Disorder (ADHD)

The clinical literature contains many descriptions of problems involving attention deficits, impulsivity, and excessive motor activity. These problems often were referred to early on as hyperkinesis or hyperactivity, but are now thought to comprise a condition of attention-deficit hyperactivity disorder (ADHD). The major characteristics or "symptoms" of ADHD (developmentally inappropriate attention span and excessive motor activity) are not always linked, but the frequency of association has led to the use of the term ADHD to refer to this complex of problems. The condition is more common in boys than in girls, is identifiable early in life, and is often associated with behavioral and learning problems. It is important to stress that ADHD and learning disabilities are not the same, because learning disabilities may exist without hyperactivity, and not all children with ADHD have learning disabilities. The conditions often co-occur or overlap, and some researchers suggest that as many as 30% of the children receiving special education services in programs for learning disabled are actually ADHD.

Despite the somewhat confusing clinical picture, there is agreement that extreme overactivity and attentional problems are recognizable in the preschool years and that they represent an early warning sign of possible problems, including learning disabilities. Campbell, Szumowski, Ewing, Gluck, and Breaux (1982) found that the "core symptoms" of inattentiveness, hyperactivity, and aggression, were identifiable by parents of 2- to 3-year-olds as well as by laboratory measures. Other researchers report that teachers also are able to identify preschool children who show signs of hyperactivity and distractibility. Inventories and rating scales such as the Conners Rating Scales (Conners, 1973) and the ADD-H Comprehensive Teacher Rating Scale (Ullmann, Sleator, & Sprague, 1985) often are used to gather adults' perceptions of children's activity level and attentional characteristics.

The ability to modulate activity level, to come to attention, to focus, and to sustain attention, are all important attributes in children's learning. These are the attributes that appear most affected in children with ADHD, and that are often found in young children with learning disabilities. Thus, they may be useful early indicators of problems.

Behavior Problems

Behavior problems, especially aggression, frequently are associated with hyperactivity, and often are viewed as predictors of later problems. The diagnostic significance of behavior problems for learning disabilities is not entirely clear, yet serious problems in socialization and behavioral control suggest possible underlying processing difficulties. Numerous checklists or inventories of problem behaviors are available for assessing behavior problems (e.g., the Child Behavior Checklist-Preschool Form, Achenbach, Edelbrock, & Howell, 1987; the Preschool Behavior Questionnaire, Behar & Stringfield, 1974). Although we usually think of behavior problems as being externalizing in nature, as characterized by aggressiveness, unruliness, and resistance to discipline, there is some indication that internalizing problems, such as withdrawal and excessive shyness, also may be associated with learning problems. In a recent meta-analysis of 58 studies, for example, Horn and Packard (1986) found that after distractibility, internalizing problem behavior was one of the best early predictors of reading failure.

It is difficult to draw definitive conclusions about direct causal relationships between behavior problems in the preschool years and learning disabilities. There are, however, some generalizations that follow from a sizeable research literature. Behavior problems may be identified reliably in the preschool years. There is considerable agreement between parents' and preschool teachers' views of problems, suggesting some stability across settings. Children referred for clinical services as learning disabled often have histories of severe behavior problems in the preschool years.

A word of caution about the interpretation of behavior problems and hyperactivity/attention disorders in the preschool years relates to their prevalence in the preschool population as a whole. Overactivity and lack of sustained attention are relatively common characteristics of 2- and 3-year-olds, and tend to change with age. Some studies have suggested that as many as 20 to 30% of preschoolers display externalizing problem behaviors. Thus, the age-related aspect of these indicators must be considered when making clinical decisions about young children. Also, it is important to emphasize that problems of attention and activity, as well as behavior problems, are situationally related, and that the context, including the constraints and characteristics of the environment, come into play. This is especially important to remember when most of the descriptions of preschool children come from reports of parents or of teachers.

Neurodevelopmental Indicators

Neurodevelopmental indicators often are used to identify preschoolers at risk for subsequent learning disabilities. Much of the early work on learning disabilities was based on the assumption of minimal brain dysfunction, and there is current research suggesting a relationship between neuromaturational indices and learning problems. Neurological "soft signs" usually include such specifics as fine and gross motor coordination problems, abnormal or choreiform movements, reflex asymmetries, and/or visual-motor abnormalities. There is also a likely overlap with ADHD, because both attention and activity problems may be considered primary (neurologically based) handicapping conditions (cf. Chapter 1). In general, hyperactivity and attentional problems are more powerful predictors of subsequent learning problems than are the neurological "soft signs." Yet, neurological symptoms may serve as "red flags" for a range of problem conditions, including learning disabilities.

The interest in neurological indicators has led to the use of a variety of tests or measures, some included in neurodevelopmental examinations (Chapter 3), others more psychologically (Chapter 4) or educationally (Chapter 5) focussed. Educationally or psychologically focussed tests are aimed at behavioral expressions of possible neurological conditions, and commonly tap perceptual and motor abilities. Widely used techniques require children to copy or reproduce designs or geometric forms, to solve maze puzzles, or to perform task requiring visual-motor coordination. As with other techniques, an important question when identifying preschool children with learning disabilities has to do with the predictive power of these tasks. In general the associations between specific signs and subsequent learning disabilities are low. Few, if any, single signs are in and of themselves powerful diagnostic indicators. On the other hand, both the "soft" neurological signs and the behavioral indicators may be part of a pattern which suggests increased vulnerability or risk for the development of learning disabilities.

APPLYING A DISCREPANCY MODEL TO PRESCHOOL IDENTIFICATION

Delays of neurodevelopment (especially language), deficits of attention, and behavior problems are all indicators of possible learning disabilities in young children. Parents and teachers need to be sensitive to delays or peculiarities in speech, to short attention span, and to persistent uncontrolled behavior outbursts. Whether these signs are specific to learning disabilities is uncertain, because in the preschool years they also may be associated with other problem conditions such as mild retardation or emotional problems. However, they send a message that some children may be "at risk" and that special attention is needed. They also are particularly useful areas to assess when diagnosing learning disabilities, because these domains represent pre-academic skills, and can be used in a discrepancy model of identification. That is, children's level of development in a specific domain, such as language or behavior, may be compared to their general level of cognitive development. In addition, assessment of children's performance in a number of pre-academic areas allows determination of discrepant patterns of development, thus providing information analogous to the achievement discrepancies in older children with learning disabilities.

Assessing Cognitive Development

Thanks to a long tradition of psychometric efforts, there are numerous well-constructed and well-studied tests that have been developed for assessing the general ability of young children. These include the Wechsler Preschool and Primary Scale of Intelligence—Revised (Wechsler, 1989), the Stanford-Binet Intelligence Scale: 4th Edition (Thorndike, Hagen, & Sattler, 1986), the McCarthy Scales of Children's Abilities (McCarthy, 1972), and the Kaufman Assessment Battery for Children (Kaufman, 1983). These scales have been normed on large samples of children and have good reliability and validity. They meet the technical requirements for tests as defined by the U.S. Office of Education Special Education Programs Work Group on Management Issues in Assessment of Learning Disabilities (Reynolds, 1984). They also have been used widely in clinical and educational assessment. These tests, in addition to developmental scales such as the Bayley Scale, the Gesell Developmental Schedules, and the Minnesota Child Development Inventory, provide ways to estimate general cognitive or developmental levels. Thus, they address one component in the discrepancy model for identifying young children with learning disabilities.

Assessing Specific Skills

Assessment of specific abilities or aptitudes of preschoolers, the other component in the discrepancy model, is not quite as clear, however. This is in part a measurement problem, as many preschool tests do not meet the technical criteria necessary for accurate assessment, although they may have "face validity." We examined 98 educationally relevant tests listed in the *Ninth Mental Measurement Yearbook* (Mitchell, 1985) as appropriate for assessment of kindergarten or preschool children. We found that many were group rather than individually administered, a large number did not provide standardized norms, some were ratings or observations rather than direct measures of skills, a few were developed for specific populations and were narrow in scope, and some were inadequately standardized with questionable reliability and validity. Our review suggests the need for careful selection of tests of specific aptitudes when diagnosing learning disabilities in preschool children, as inappropriate or unreliable measurement is a threat to accuracy when used in the discrepancy model.

In general, two main types of procedures are used in assessing young children: rating scales and direct assessment/testing. Both are based on the assumptions that there are early indicators that are valid predictors of subsequent learning disabilities; and, that those indicators can be identified and measured reliably. As noted earlier, although many of the scales and tests have good face validity and tap child characteristics that seem logical and sensible, solid evidence documenting predictive validity or accuracy is limited. However, despite potential problems and limitations, both ratings and direct assessment are useful. Several examples of well-known scales and tests have been selected for illustrative purposes.

Rating Scales

The number of published rating scales attests to their utility and popularity. Many are aimed at gathering information from parents, teachers, or others close to the children being studied. Scales tap a range of child characteristics, some focussing on specific pre-academic behaviors and aptitudes, others covering a broad range of content. The Preschool Behavior Questionnaire (Behar & Stringfield, 1974) is aimed specifically at identifying emotional/behavioral problems in children 3 to 6 years of age. Teachers or child-care workers are asked to rate children on 36 items tapping three domains: anxious-fearful, hyperactive-distractible, and hostile-aggressive. The Revised Behavior Problem Checklist (1987) contains items appropriate for children ages 5 to 12 years, and consists of 89 items to be rated by teachers or parents. The scale yields six scores: conduct disorder, socialized aggression, attention problems and immaturity, anxiety-withdrawal, and psychotic behavior.

Some rating scales used for screening are focussed more specifically on school-related learning and classroom behaviors. The Rhode Island Profile of Early Learning Behavior (1982) is a 40-item scale to be completed by classroom teachers, kindergarten to Grade 2. The ratings yield scores about classroom behavior, written work, and a total score. The Pupil Rating Scale-Revised: Screening for Learning Disabilities (1981) was designed to gather teachers' and counselors' views of children 5 to 14 years of age. The kindergarten to Grade 6 form consists of 24 items tapping verbal and nonverbal skills, auditory comprehension and memory, spoken language, and motor coordination.

In addition to published rating scales of the kinds just described, many scales have been developed within school districts or for particular research projects. When used by professionals who have had an opportunity to become well acquainted with children, many of these rating scales have been found to be effective in identifying children with learning problems. However, whether standardized and published or locally developed and unique, all rating instruments must be evaluated in terms of their predictive validity and appropriateness. Issues of reliability of measurement must be considered, especially when ratings provide the basis for placement or instructional decisions. Professionals' expectations, attitudes, values, and prior experiences may bias their ratings and lead to erroneous decisions regarding a child's status as at risk for learning disabilities. On the positive side, parents and teachers who work with children on a daily basis are an important and useful source of information, and may well serve as the "first screen" in identifying young children with learning disabilities.

Direct Assessment

The second main approach to identification involves direct assessment of specific skills, and there are many published tests and procedures for this purpose. As with rating scales, tests differ in focus and scope, in technical and psychometric adequacy, and in predictive validity. They also differ in administrative time and conditions and in cost. Some may be administered to groups of children, others require individual administration; some assess a broad range of child abilities, others are aimed at identification of specific problems, for example, neurological "soft signs" or language delays. The Boehm Test of Basic Concepts, designed for use with children in kindergarten to Grade 2, covers children's understanding of 50 "basic concepts" such as quantity or time. The concepts tested are important for school success, but seem to tap general cognitive skills rather than specific precursors of academic subjects. A similar concern may be raised about the Brigance Preschool Screen, an assessment technique approach for 3-year-old children. The screen assesses basic readiness skills and development, but with a few exceptions, does not assess specific academic preskills. The Slingerland Pre-Reading Screening Procedures Revised (1980), administered to children individually, assess entering school children's abilities on 12 dimensions thought to be related to reading (e.g., visual and auditory skills, auditory-visual association). The Development Indicators for the Assessment of Learning-Revised (DIAL-R) (1983) is an individually administered screening test aimed at identifying children at risk for learning problems at or before school entrance. The test yields motor, concepts, language, and total scores. Both the Slingerland Procedures and the DIAL-R are lengthy and require a minimum of 30 to 40 minutes to administer.

Other screening tests are focussed on specific ability areas such as language, mathematics, or reading. The Test of Early Language Development (TELD) (1981) or the revised Test of Language Development-Primary (TOLD-P) (1982) are examples of individually administered tests designed to screen for problems in receptive and/or expressive language. Group screening measures are also available and often used. The Comprehensive Test of Basic Skills (1981, 1982, 1983) and the Metropolitan Achievement Tests (1984) are well known group readiness tests that are designed to yield information about children's competencies or problems in both language and quantitative areas. The content of possible screening tests is broad, and there also is variation in their technical adequacy. Thus, effective and accurate early identification requires careful selection of methods and instruments and appropriate and sensitive implementation procedures.

Influences of Children's Performance on Tests

Although many tests may have good technical or psychometric properties, numerous other factors may influence children's performance, and thus, may distort early identification findings. Possible challenges to the validity of results range from the obvious to the subtle, but, nonetheless, all need to be taken into account when planning and implementing programs for early identification of children who are learning disabled.

Two points are particularly important when testing children. The first has to do with the language and cultural background of children being assessed. Non- or limited-English speaking children, or children whose home language is dialect based, are clearly at a disadvantage when test material is presented in standard English. Some tests are nonverbal in content and do not require spoken answers and are considered "non-language." However, there are many linguistic demands in most tests, including nonverbal tasks, which may distort or reduce children's responses. In addition, cultural difference in interaction styles, in children's behavioral styles, may interfere with their performance in a testing setting, lowering their scores and leading to incorrect inferences about their cognitive abilities or their readiness for school. Gandara, Keogh, and Yoshioka-Maxwell (1980) tested the predictive validity of several screening measures, including a nonlanguage Piagetian approach, with Anglo and Hispanic kindergarten children. Not surprisingly, all methods were accurate predictors of subsequent school performance for Anglo children. However, none of the measures was accurate in predicting first grade achievement for the Spanish-speaking Hispanic children. We must, then, question the use of many conventional tests for assessing children from nonmajority language and cultural backgrounds.

In addition, it is assumed that children come to the testing situation with similar and necessary experiences, and that they have the prerequisite background to perform. Thus, when performance is poor it can be inferred that some deficits in cognition, attention, language, or other ability domains are present. The assumption of prerequisite skills may be inaccurate in many cases, and indeed, there is evidence that poor performance sometimes may be related to lack of experience with the materials and demands of the tests themselves. Dreisbach and Keogh (1982) trained Hispanic, Spanish-speaking children in test-taking skills (e.g., "Here is what it means to put a circle around the answer," "This is how you underline the answer"). They found that the trained children significantly outperformed the nontrained children on a standard readiness test, although there was nothing in the brief training sessions that dealt with content. These findings suggest that experience in school-like activities, including test-taking skills, affect children's performance on tests, so that poor scores may be related to lack of experience rather than to general or specific deficits or delays. This, of course, infers the need to exercise caution when attributing poor scores to child deficits.

ADDITIONAL DIAGNOSTIC CRITERIA

Useful diagnostic information also is gained from understanding not just what a child does or does not do, but how, how often, and under what conditions the problem behaviors occur. Information relevant to these criteria is not gathered necessarily from tests or direct assessment of children, but may be gleaned from interviews with parents and teachers and from naturalistic observations of children. Parents and teachers may learn a great deal about problem behaviors by keeping a log or diary which documents misbehaviors and the circumstances in which they occur. Such information allows evaluation of the behavior in terms of intensity, chronicity, breadth, and stability.

Severity or intensity of a problem behavior is of real concern, and adults usually are well aware of this aspect of a problem. All preschoolers have outbursts of frustration and temper and may have episodes of sulking or withdrawal; most preschool children are physically active. The intensity of expression will vary, however, and some behaviors go considerably beyond expected bounds. Inappropriately intense or severe misbehavior, thus, may be an indication of learning problems.

Closely related, the frequency of expression or the regularity of problem behavior also is useful diagnostic information. Occasional inappropriate, ineffective, or maladaptive behaviors are to be expected in preschool children. Young children are learning new skills, are trying out new strategies; it is not surprising that their efforts are sometimes discrepant or disruptive. When such behaviors occur frequently or typically, however, they suggest a lack of adequate coping skills, and may be signals of problems.

Particular behaviors also need to be evaluated relative to the settings or situations in which they occur, as the diagnostic significance of a particular behavior is related to its breadth of expression. Is the behavior evident in many situations or is it situation-specific? Is the child overly active at home and at school? When playing with friends or with adults? Maladaptive or negative behaviors which are evident in only one situation likely are not as serious as behaviors that are evident across a range of settings and across many learning tasks.

Finally, the stability of problem behaviors over time is another important diagnostic indicator. The preschool years are a time of rapid change, and problem behaviors early on often are replaced by more adaptive and mature skills, so that many behavior or learning problems are transitory. A 2-year-old may have brief periods of difficulty in sustaining attention so that he or she appears distractible and impulsive. A 3-year-old may stammer or reverse words for a few weeks or months. These are not necessarily signs of learning disabilities, but may represent transition periods in development or be responses to stress. On the other hand, a learning disability may be suggested if the same behaviors or indicators are maintained over long periods of time and if they are not replaced by more effective and age-appropriate behaviors.

CONCLUSION

Identifying children with learning disabilities in the preschool years is not just a matter of testing, although there are a number of instruments and behavior surveys that are useful identification procedures. Rather, sensitive and accurate identification of young children with learning disabilities requires consideration of the severity, chronicity, breadth, and stability of problems. Evaluating behaviors and problems within a developmental perspective ensures an age- and gender-appropriate framework. A developmental perspective provides the background for determining discrepancies in general aptitude and specific skills and for identifying uneven patterns of growth that are characteristics of children with learning disabilities. Thus, it allows identification of young children with learning disabilities using a model consistent with the discrepancy model employed with school-age children.

Finally, and perhaps most important, when working with preschool children, we must view early identification of learning disabilities as *tentative*. Young children are remarkably resilient, and given timely and appropriate help, many young children with learning disabilities develop into competent and successful students. The importance of early identification is that it allows parents and teachers to provide the help necessary to achieve those goals.

CHAPTER 3

Neurodevelopmental Evaluation (The Physician's Diagnostic Role in Learning Disabilities)

Frank R. Brown, III

The diagnosis of learning disabilities for school-age children has traditionally depended upon measurement of, and establishment of, a discrepancy between academic achievement and cognitive functioning levels. In Chapter 2 we noted some of the difficulties in using discrepancy definitions to identify preschool-age children at risk for subsequent learning disabilities, and we discussed the utility of a neurodevelopmental/behavioral approach to facilitate early identification of children at risk for subsequent poor academic achievement. The physician plays a vital role in the interdisciplinary approach to identification and remediation of learning disabilities. In the case of preschool-age children, the physician frequently is the first professional resource consulted regarding questions of neurodevelopmental/behavioral progress. When questions arise about learning disabilities in school-age children, the physician can contribute both in the diagnostic process and in ensuring a balance of professional perspectives when establishing a remediation program. To make these contributions to the diagnostic and prescriptive process for both preschool and school-age children, the physician must expand the traditional role of medical history taking and examination to include a *neurodevelopmental history* and *neurodevelopmental examination*. Components of the physician's expanded neurodevelopmental history and examination process for the preschool and school-age child are the focus of this chapter.

IDENTIFICATION OF PRESCHOOL-AGE CHILDREN AT RISK FOR LEARNING DISABILITIES

Unfortunately, there does not yet exist a reliable method for identifying children with learning disabilities at an early age (before first grade, and usually not until beginning second grade). One approach to early identification of preschool-age children "at risk" for subsequent learning disabilities is to identify patterns of neurodevelopment that correlate with subsequent learning difficulties, looking especially for delays in language understanding and usage, visual perception, attention and/or impulse control, and for the presence of any associated oppositional, noncompliant, and avoidant behaviors. The physician has a vital role to play in this approach to early identification, and the physician's assessment begins with the neurodevelopmental history.

Neurodevelopmental History

The neurodevelopmental history, that is, the history of the temporal sequence of development, is an important element of the physician's evaluation of the preschool child at risk for subsequent learning disabilities. The importance and utility of the neurodevelopmental history is underscored by the following elements.

1. The neurodevelopmental history affords the physician multiple "windows" on the course of neurodevelopment to date. Consistencies observed within the neurodevelopmental history and between the history and neurodevelopmental examination improve reliability and validity of conclusions regarding levels of neurodevelopmental function.

2. The neurodevelopmental history affords the physician an opportunity to compare present and past rates of neurodevelopment. Such comparisons assist the physician in determining whether developmental delays manifest as a constant, albeit slower than normal rate of development or as a progressive deterioration in neurodevelopment ("progressive encephalopathy" or "neurodegenerative disorder").

3. The neurodevelopmental history can assist the physician in determining what, if any, additional diagnostic tests to perform. A history suggesting a constant, albeit slower than normal rate of development may disincline the physician from performing elaborate studies to establish causation. The yield of such efforts, both from the standpoint

of establishing causation and from the standpoint of identifying treatable disorders, is usually limited. On the other hand, a history consistent with neurodegeneration should alert the physician to perform a variety of additional diagnostic tests, for example, computer assisted tomography, nuclear magnetic resonance scans, electroencephalograms, urine metabolic screens, serum and urinary amino acid screens, biochemical evaluations of cultured skin fibroblasts. By restricting use of these diagnostic studies to those progressive neurological processes identified in the neurodevelopmental history, the physician can optimally identify those children whose course is expected to be altered by this information.

4. The neurodevelopmental history affords the physician a temporal accounting of developmental progress, and can serve as a guideline to the appropriate level at which to begin the neurodevelopmental examination.

5. Comparison of the parents' accounting of the neurodevelopmental history with developmental findings observed in the neurodevelopmental examination affords the physician and interdisciplinary team insight into how realistic the parents are in their understanding of the extent of their child's problems. This information can help guide subsequent parent conferences and counseling sessions.

The first part of the neurodevelopmental history is the ascertainment of any pre- and/or perinatal risk factors (Table 3-1) that might place the child at increased risk for subsequent developmental disabilities, including specific learning disabilities. The physician and interdisciplinary team must appreciate that many affected children may not have obvious histories of pre- and/or perinatal risk factors. In fact, although a significant number of children with a high risk pre- or perinatal course will manifest subsequent neurological deficits, the majority of children with neurological deficits do not have histories that we would identify as high risk. This may reflect the fact that many of the risk factors listed in Table 3-1 can manifest in subtle, sometimes undetectable fashion, and/or that current technologies are not sophisticated enough to detect more subtle insults. For example, although the effects of high maternal alcohol consumption on the fetus and full-blown fetal alcohol syndrome are obvious (intrauterine and postnatal growth retardation, physical abnormalities, and impaired cognitive development), the effects of lesser degrees of alcohol and cigarette consumption, as well as other factors such as subclinical maternal viral infections on the developing fetus are less obvious. Certainly the presence of risk factors in the pregnancy, labor, and delivery should alert the physician to carefully monitor subsequent neurodevelopment. We hope in the future

TABLE 3-1

Prenatal and Perinatal History—Risk Factors Associated with Learning Disabilities

Pregnancy	Labor and Delivery (cont'd)
Maternal age	Problems:
Paternal age	premature rupture of membranes
Parity	maternal fever
Length of gestation	toxemia
Maternal weight gain	abnormal bleeding
Fetal activity	fetal monitoring
Previous maternal obstetrical problems	failure of labor to progress
	labor induced
Problems:	Caesarian section
bleeding/spotting	forceps/instrumentation
medications	resuscitation
trauma	abnormalities at birth
toxemia	abnormal placenta
radiation	**Neonatal**
rash/infection	
fluid retention	Duration of hospitalization
abnormal fetal movements	Problems:
alcohol	respiratory distress syndrome
tobacco	cyanosis
Labor and Delivery	seizures
Hospital	oxygen therapy
Duration of labor	feeding problems
Birth weight	infections
Apgars	jaundice
Analgesia/sedation	metabolic
Presentation	congenital abnormalities
	apnea

that the ability to identify milder (and more frequently occurring) insults will improve.

In addition to the historical questions used to identify high risk pre- and perinatal situations, the physician should elicit a careful neurodevelopmental history, that is, a history of temporal development in four areas:

1. Motor—including gross, fine, and oral motor function.
2. Visual perception and problem solving-including concepts such as size, shape, and spatial relationships.
3. Language—including expressive and receptive language abilities.

4. Social-adaptive—including self-help skills such as dressing and feeding.

As the physician elicits the temporal sequence of development in these four areas, it is important that he or she be cognizant of the fact that parents frequently have difficulty recalling neurodevelopment in those areas in which the physician has most interest, especially receptive language and visual perception/problem solving. Parents usually have an easier time relaying historical information regarding events that they perceive as major events in their child's life (e.g., age at which the child took his or her first step or uttered first words). As the physician initiates the neurodevelopmental history, it is advisable that he or she build the parents' confidence as historians by asking them to recount their child's development in those areas where they are anticipated to be the best observers. In most instances this proves to be gross motor (Table 3-2) and expressive language development (Table 3-3) (i.e., "walking" and "talking"). After building the parents' confidence in their ability to recall historical details, the physician can proceed to elicit the neurodevelopmental history in those important, but more difficult areas to recall, such as receptive language (Table 3-3) and visual perception/problem solving (Table 3-4).

TABLE 3-2
Gross Motor Developmental Milestones

Approximate Age	Skill Attained
4 mo	Roll over, face down to face up
5 mo	Roll over, face up to face down
6 mo	Sit without support
9 mo	Pull to standing
12 mo	Walk independently
18 mo	Run
27 mo	Walk up stairs ("marking time")
36 mo	Walk up stairs alternating feet and down stairs ("marking time")
	Pedal tricycle
3.5 yr	Walk up and down stairs alternating feet
5 yr	Skip
7 yr	Ride two-wheel bicycle without training wheels

Because the parents will not be as accurate in recalling details regarding receptive language and visual perception/problem solving, the physician sometimes will have to be creative and persistent in the history-taking process, asking questions in a proper sequence to maximize accuracy of the parents' recollections. For example, questions regarding visual perception need to be asked in a fashion that the parents appreciate, that is, in terms of tasks that relate to everyday living. This approach might mean that visual perception would be evaluated through a history of development of skills such as dressing and feeding, skills that depend on a combination of visual perception and problem solving. Such items also represent "social-adaptive" development, and

TABLE 3-3
Language—Expressive and Receptive

Approximate Age	Skill Attained
6 mo	Babbling (playful repetition of consonant-vowel syllables—should consist of at least four different consonants repeated in a string)
9 mo	Gesture language (child either spontaneously or imitatively engages in gestures to communicate wants; waves bye-bye or plays pat-a-cake)
12 mo	Ma-Ma/Da-Da, used appropriately to mean mother or father
	First word other than ma-ma, da-da, or name of family member
18 mo	Follow one-step command without gestures, (e.g., "Give me _____")
2 yr	Two word phrases, 20 word vocabulary
2.5 yr	Follows two-step command without gestures, (e.g., "Put the ball on the table and give the pencil to me")
3 yr	Vocabulary 250 words, three- and four-word sentences
	Answers appropriately, "What do you do when you are hungry?"
4 yr	Tells stories about experiences using complex syntax
	Answers appropriately, "What is a house made of?"
5 yr	Vocabulary too numerous to count
	Follows three-step command in the correct order

NEURODEVELOPMENTAL EVALUATION

depend heavily on fine motor development, as well as on the parents' willingness to allow the child to express developmental capabilities.

The physician should conclude the neurodevelopmental history by asking the parents to state their perceptions of their child's overall level of neurodevelopmental function—stated in terms of age equivalents. This question can be as simple as "At what age level do you see your

TABLE 3-4

Assessment of Visual Problem-Solving Abilities

One-Inch Cubes (18 months to 7 years)

18 mo	Vertical tower of 3 cubes (a)	(a)
24 mo	Train of 3 cubes (b)	(b)
27 mo	Train of 4 cubes with smoke stack (c)	(c)
36 mo	3 block bridge (d)	(d)
4 yr	5 block gate (e)	(e)
5 yr	6 block staircase (f)	(f)
7 yr	10 block staircase (g)	(g)

Pencil and Paper (3 to 12 years)

3 yr	Copies circle
3.5 yr	Copies cross
4 yr	Copies square
5 yr	Copies triangle
6 yr	Copies "Union Jack"
7 yr	Copies diamond
8 yr	Copies Maltese cross
9 yr	Copies cylinder
12 yr	Copies cube

Gesell Drawings (see Figure 3-1)

child functioning overall?" If the parents show any resistance in formulating a response, they should be further encouraged to "Give me your best guess." If both parents are present, the question should be asked separately to determine concurrence (this concurrence may be of import later during the parent conference). Further clarification is afforded if the parents are asked to describe age equivalents for areas of "best function" and "worst function." Parents' willingness and concurrence in estimating an age-equivalent of their child's development may indicate the degree to which parents will be able to accept later diagnostic formulations. In addition, the physician may find that parents are better able to accept diagnostic conclusions if they have initially acknowledged that their child is delayed in one or more areas.

The physician should resist simple conclusions that parents are "poor" or "bad" historians, and rather make a concerted effort to become a more effective history taker. "Bad" historians, meaning parents who provide misinformation because of unpreparedness to accept their own suspicions of delay, are extremely rare. Numerous factors can contribute to a poor history-taking process. When a child exhibits significant delays in an area of neurodevelopmental function, not only will development of the process be protracted over time (and therefore its precise time of evolution be somewhat blurred), but also the quality of the process will be affected, and therefore the parents may have difficulty recalling specific ages of attainment. The physician also should be careful to avoid the perception by the parents that he or she views the child's neurodevelopment as a rote compendium of deficits. The physician should develop the history via questions focussed exclusively on age-equivalent descriptors, for example, "At what age did your child walk independently?" The physician should avoid questions that imply perceptions of delay, for example, "When did you appreciate your child's delay in walking?" Terms that imply delayed development, such as "slow," "delayed," or "disabled" should be assiduously avoided because they afford miscommunication. These summary descriptors serve no purpose other than to potentially offend and distort the history-taking process.

Having obtained estimates of current neurodevelopmental functioning (i.e., age equivalents) through the neurodevelopmental history, the physician will progress to the second component of the physician's process, the neurodevelopmental examination. If the history and examination are performed properly, the examination should simply confirm levels of neurodevelopmental function inferred in the history, and the combination of the two will produce a reliable and valid assessment.

Neurodevelopmental Examination

Physicians typically have utilized "screening instruments" as a basis for neurodevelopmental examination and in making decisions regarding referrals for more detailed evaluations. Reliance on any single screening instrument is problematic for the following reasons:

1. These instruments often result in significant false positives and negatives, and referral decisions based on them are apt to be inaccurate.
2. Their design and use affords a limited perspective on neurodevelopment, that is, at only one point in time. This contrasts with and ignores the important utility of the developmental history and leads to the false positives and negatives described previously.
3. Their design affords no reliability or validity of observation unless another instrument is administered.
4. Overreliance on screening instruments translates into "test scores" with poor appreciation of the process utilized by the generalist in looking at neurodevelopment.

We feel that assessment and referral decisions regarding preschool-age children at risk for subsequent learning disabilities are best made on the basis of appreciation of normal and abnormal development, the depth and breadth of training of the physician, and the reliability and validity inherent in the neurodevelopmental history and examination gathering process. The neurodevelopmental assessment tools described are not intended to replace more detailed evaluations by allied health professionals, but they can help the generalist develop appropriate schema for subsequent referrals.

The neurodevelopmental examination is the physician's detailed examination of a child's development in the four areas discussed previously: motor (gross/fine/oral), visual perception and problem solving, language (expressive/receptive), and social-adaptive function. Social-adaptive function, for example, self-help skills such as dressing and feeding, usually is not directly assessed in the neurodevelopmental examination because of time constraints and lack of efficiency.

Because the child's cooperation is essential for accurate assessment of cognitive function, and because cognitive function is deemed to be particularly germane to prediction of future school success, we recommend that the neurodevelopmental examination of the preschool-age child commence with cognitive assessment and proceed subsequently to analysis of motor skills. We recommend initiating cognitive assessment with visual perceptual problem solving, then proceeding to language. A good reason for conducting the examination in this order is to guard against the child who may have disproportionate delay in language functioning relative to other cognitive abilities. This approach is particularly advised when the parents' neurodevelopmental history suggests that such problems in language exist. It is our experience that if such children are approached initially with any significant language demand, that further cooperation in the examining process will be impaired. Rapport will, of course, be further enhanced by careful selection of initial areas and levels of assessment so as to avoid challenging the child in areas of relative weakness.

Assessment of Visual Perceptual/Problem-Solving Abilities

Assessment of visual problem solving for preschool-age children involves analysis of play-like skills with simple toy items of the type described in Table 3-4. Many of these test items are high-interest tasks and similar to children's play. As a result, for many children, visual problem solving is an ideal starting point in the neurodevelopmental examination. Assessment of visual problem solving for children is dependent upon a combination of the cognitive ability to visually conceptualize the task, as well as the fine motor skill to respond. The interdependency of these two processes points up the need to dissociate inability to perform a task into its requisite parts.

Several of the toy items used to assess visual problem solving, especially one-inch cubes and pencil or crayons and paper, cover a fairly broad range of developmental abilities. The one-inch cubes, for example, cover a visual perceptual/fine motor neurodevelopmental age range of approximately 3 months to 7 years, and pencil or crayons and paper an approximate 16 months to 12 year range. Because they are useful in assessment of visual perception/visual problem solving across such a breadth of developmental age range, and because they represent very simple test procedures that the physician may incorporate in the neurodevelopmental assessment battery, these two items have particular utility.

When assessing a child's visual perceptual abilities with one-inch cubes, the examiner first builds the block constructs out of the child's field of view (typically by covering the assembly process with the examiner's hand). The child is then given the appropriate number of blocks to build a duplicate of the examiner's model, and the model is left in place for visual imitation by the child. The two exceptions to this procedure are the staircase assemblies (Table 3-4, f and g), where the model is built out of sight, shown to the child, and destroyed, and the child is then asked to build the assembly from visual memory.

The drawing tasks listed in Table 3-4 are suitable for testing visual perceptual development over a wide age range. The Gesell figures (Figure 3-1) are a series of increasingly complex figures that the child is asked to replicate with crayon or pencil and paper. These drawings are presented to the child in a completed, predrawn fashion and the child is asked to draw a likeness of the figures. It is imperative that the physician observe the child in the process of replicating the figures, as satisfactory replication is not the only information to be obtained. Rather it is important to analyze the child's approach to replication of the figures, including issues such as time to complete the figures and omission of key elements. The child who does not understand the gestalt of the figures may, for example, approach the "Union Jack" in a fragmented fashion, perhaps drawing it as a series of small triangles. Unless the child is observed in the drawing process these qualitative deficits in performance may not be appreciated.

Assessment of Language Functioning

As discussed earlier, several aspects of neurodevelopmental function in the preschool-age child are particularly suggestive that a child is at increased risk for subsequent learning difficulties. Of all neurodevelopmental domains, receptive language is perhaps most predictive of future developmental course. Particular attention should be paid to elucidation of the neurodevelopmental history and in neurodevelopmental assessment in this domain.

Assessment of language functioning does not depend on specific test items of the type described for assessment of visual perceptual abilities. When assessing language development in the preschool-age child, the examiner should be most concerned with connected language understanding and usage. This most meaningful aspect of the preschooler's language development can be assessed simply and appropriately by examination of ability to manipulate familiar objects upon command (i.e., follow simple directions, with and without gestures and of increasing complexity) and ability to answer simple comprehension questions exemplified in Table 3-3. Instruments such as the Peabody Picture Vocabulary Test-Revised (PPVT-R) assess more limited aspects of language development (picture identification), and therefore are less informative of meaningful language development. In other words, the generalist might well attach more meaning to the child's ability to comprehend the direction "put the book in the drawer" (an approximate 30 months of age task), than the ability to identify pictures in the book (PPVT-R).

An important "red flag" in identifying language delay is the persistence of echolalia beyond approximately 30 months of age. Echolalia,

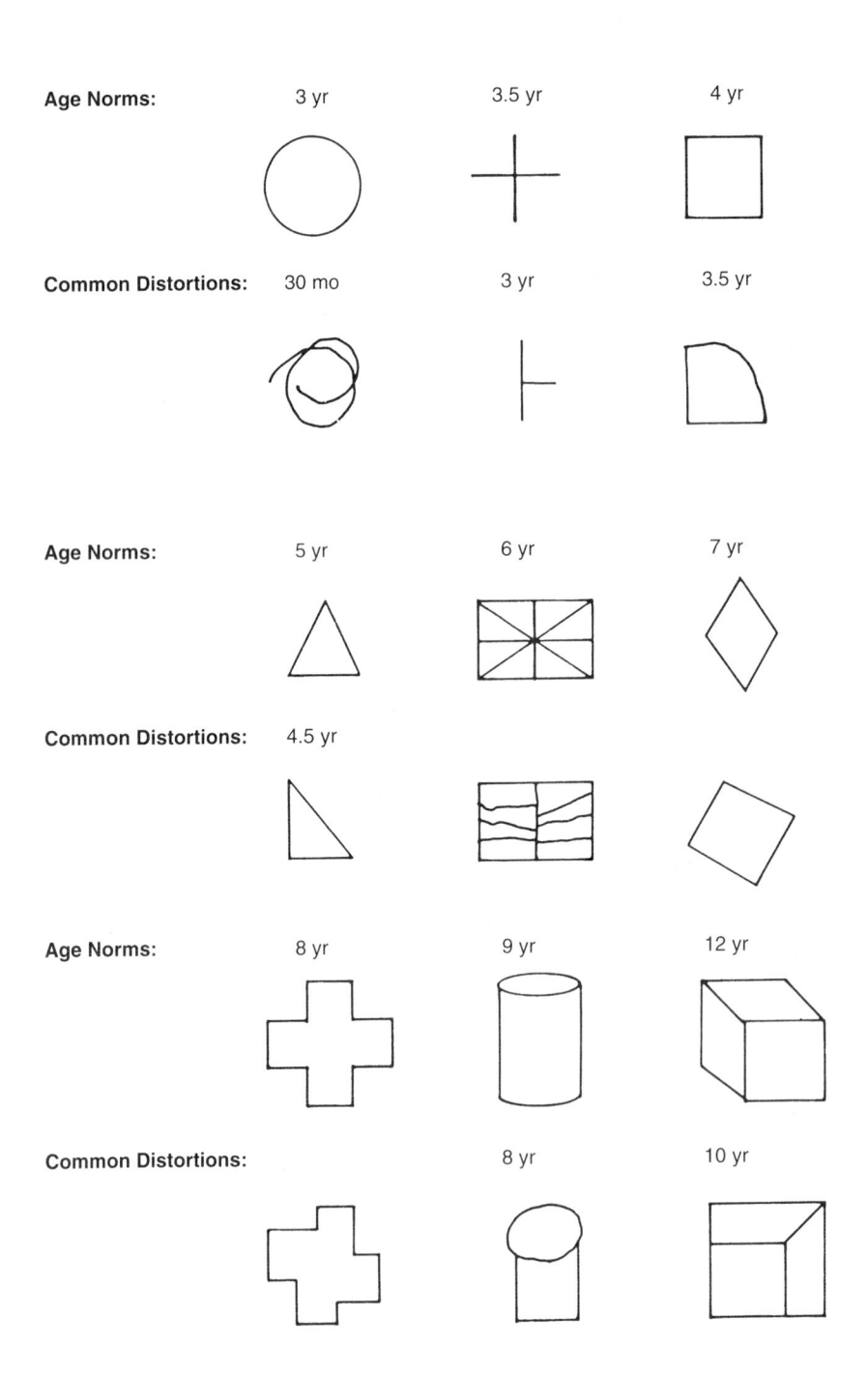

FIGURE 3-1. *Assessment of Visual Problem-Solving Abilities (Gesell Drawings)*

46

as exemplified by the repetition of a question rather than responding to the question, or echoing the last thing heard (e.g., Question: "Are you a boy or a girl?" Answer: "boy or girl"), represents a failure to comprehend language. Presence of echolalia beyond 30 months of age is tantamount to saying that the child is delayed in the language sphere.

Within the context of an office setting it is unrealistic to expect a child to exhibit a reasonable facsimile of his or her expressive vocabulary and mean length of utterance. To estimate expressive language the examiner will have to rely in significant part on the parents' history. This need not be a major deterrent to assessment of expressive language, as long as the examiner is cognizant of the fact that it is impossible for receptive language to lag expressive language development. On the other hand, expressive language, at least in the usual restricted evaluative setting, may well appear to lag receptive language development. Receptive language is, therefore, usually considered a far better indicator of inherent language capabilities.

Assessment of Gross/Fine/Oral Motor Abilities

Having completed the cognitive (visual perceptual and language assessment) portion of the neurodevelopmental examination, the examiner will proceed with assessment of motor function. This domain is reserved for the last part of the examination because it represents a more invasive aspect of the examination process, that is, the child is actually approached physically. In addition, it is more effective to assess cognitive domains before the child becomes tired, and it is more likely that the physician can continue to elicit cooperation in motor tasks that may be perceived as fun.

The gross motor milestones listed in Table 3-2 can be used as a guideline for examination of gross motor development in the preschool-age child. It is important to appreciate that many gross motor skills, for example ability to sit independently and to function in sitting, are attained over significant intervals of time. Children normally develop the ability to sit independently without support at approximately 6 months. Other more refined aspects of sitting may develop from 6 to 12 months of age. The ability to lateralize in sitting (i.e., ability to reach out to the side in sitting) and to exhibit a lateral protective response (i.e., the ability to catch oneself when falling to the side in sitting) normally develop at 8 months. The posterior protective response in sitting (i.e., ability to catch oneself in a rearward fall with the arms) normally emerges at 12 months of age. In summary, sitting does not develop at a single age, but rather develops at least over an age range of 6 to 12 months, and there are aspects of sitting that are still developing at a time when a child normally is beginning to walk independently.

A child's ability to perform on stairs (cf. Table 3-2) can be a tool for assessing gross motor development for children at an approximate 2.5 to 3.5 year level. At 2.5 years, a child should be able to ascend stairs with alternating feet. At 3 years, a child will ascend stairs with alternating feet and will descend stairs "marking time." Also, at about 3 years, a child normally will have developed ability to peddle a tricycle. By 3.5 years, a child will ascend and descend stairs with alternating feet.

As mentioned previously in the section on visual perceptual/fine motor assessment, an important antecedent to assessment of visual perceptual abilities is ascertainment of the extent of any intercurrent difficulties in fine motor performance. Assessment of fine motor abilities typically is inferred from observation of a child's performance on visual problem-solving tasks. An exact level of fine motor function is not derived from this process. Rather, analysis of the extent to which fine motor difficulties might represent an interfering factor is inferred.

Oral motor functioning is inferred from the neurodevelopmental history and observation in such areas as feeding and speech articulation. Certainly a history of feeding difficulties and/or persistence of drooling is suggestive of significant delays. An additional manifestation of oral motor dysfunction is delayed speech articulation. In general, children's speech should be nearly 100% intelligible to the parents by age 30 months and to strangers by 36 months.

NEURODEVELOPMENTAL HISTORY AND EXAMINATION FOR THE SCHOOL-AGE CHILD

The neurodevelopmental history and examination process described previously serves well for children under 5 years of age and permits identification of preschool children at risk for subsequent learning difficulties based on delays in neurodevelopment. When the physician is asked to evaluate school-age children for possible learning disabilities the evaluative task will be different. The physician's role in identification of preschool-age children "at risk" for subsequent learning difficulties was described as involving primarily early recognition of children with delays in neurodevelopment, especially in the areas of language understanding and usage, and visual perception/problem solving. Subsequent chapters will discuss the physician's role in early identification of developmentally inappropriate attention span and/or impulse control (Chapter 10) and behavioral disturbances including oppositional, noncompliant, and avoidant behaviors (Chapter 11).

The physician plays a role in identification of learning disabilities in school-age children by performing a neurodevelopmental evaluation that will at least screen whether discrepancies exist between cognitive expectation and academic achievement. The physician has some tools available to assess developmental functioning and academic achievement levels for these older, school-age children. However, because of the older age and the possibility of overlap with more specific testing performed by the psychologist or special educator, the physician more typically will defer to these colleagues and ask that precise levels of cognitive functioning be established on the basis of more detailed psychological and special education assessments, as described in Chapters 4 and 5. The physician evaluating the school-age child is looking for neurodevelopmental findings that, although not pathognomonic for identification of learning disabilities, nevertheless correlate quite highly with and are risk factors for subsequent development of learning disabilities.

Neurodevelopmental History

The physician's history for the school-age child with learning difficulties begins in the same format employed with the preschool child; that is, the history will begin with a review of the pregnancy, labor, and birth history to identify pregnancies that represent high risks for subsequent developmental problems (Table 3-1). The physician will next elicit a neurodevelopmental history, that is, a history of temporal patterns of development. Historical questions will be asked in the developmental areas discussed previously for the preschool child, especially detailing the parents' conception of the preschool developmental course in motor (gross/fine) and language (expressive/receptive) areas. The history to this point then identifies risk factors in the pregnancy, labor and delivery, and slowness in early (preschool) development for the child.

The remainder of the history will be somewhat similar to that elicited by the psychologist and educational specialist. Questions typically will be asked regarding present educational placement (including the current type of class and present attempts at remediation), past educational placements and attempts at remediation, the parents' conception of present levels of academic achievement and developmental (cognitive) functioning, presence of attention deficits and behavioral problems (and whether these are occurring more at home or in school), family history of learning disabilities and related developmental problems, and psychosocial circumstances of the family. A flow sheet for this history-taking process is shown in Table 3-5.

The history described previously is obtained in major part directly from the parents. Supplementary information can be obtained through

TABLE 3-5
History Taking—School-Age Child

EDUCATION—CURRENT PLACEMENT
School
Grade
Type of class
Description of specific remedial assistance
Problems:
    Academic—present academic achievement levels
    Behavior—problems occuring in school setting

BEHAVIOR
Disposition
Interpersonal relationships
Group activities
Hobbies/interests
Behavior problems:
    Short attention span
    Attention seeking
    Distractibility
    Impulsivity
    Hyperactivity
    Noncompliance
    Oppositionalism
    Avoidance
    Truancy
    Fire Setting
    Cruelty to animals
    Lying
    Stealing
Parental management of behavior

FAMILY/PSYCHOSOCIAL HISTORY
Family History (for both mother and father)
    Age
    Education
    Academic problems—including family history of learning disability
    Illness
    Occupation
    Marital Status
Social History
    Marital problems
    Caretakers
    Financial problems
    Medical insurance

phone conversations with school personnel and review of materials submitted by the school, as well as through the team staffing conference (Chapter 8). Comparison of the school's information with the parents' history can be very instructive of the depth and accuracy of the parents' understanding of issues relevant to their child's learning difficulties. This insight will be of great value in subsequent counseling with the family.

Neurodevelopmental Examination

Because of the complexities of cognitive functioning and academic achievement in school-age children, the physician does not directly assess abilities in these areas, but rather defers to colleagues in psychology and education. Similarly, language is generally assessed by the speech-language pathologist. The physician's examination of the school-age child with learning difficulties should focus on delineation of the neurodevelopmental history and examination of other neurodevelopmental factors that often are associated with learning disabilities. The physician should assess visual perceptual development (using drawing and block assembly tasks), short-term memory deficits, laterality, hand dominance, and soft neurological signs. The relationships between these factors and learning disabilities, and their utility in the remediation process remains unclear. Although deficits in these areas are not pathognomonic of learning disabilities, they frequently are observed in conjunction with learning disabilities. For that reason, the physician's assessment of these factors contributes to the diagnosis. The remainder of this chapter will focus on methods for examining performance in these areas.

Assessment of Visual Perceptual Development—Gesell Figures

There are a variety of drawing tests that may be used appropriately by the physician or allied personnel to assess visual perceptual/motor development. The Gesell figures, a series of increasingly complex figures that the child is asked to reproduce, generally represent the most useful. These drawings (Figure 3-1) are presented to the child in a completed, predrawn fashion, and the child is asked to produce a likeness of the figures. It is mandatory that the physician observe the child in the drawing process, as satisfactory completion of the drawings is not the only information to be gleaned. For example, the child with attention-deficit hyperactivity disorder (ADHD) may execute the figures in driven fashion, omitting key elements of the drawings (e.g., omission of component lines in the "Union Jack" figure). The child who does not understand the gestalt of the figures may, although producing a satisfactory final representation of the figures, assemble the drawings in an abnormal fashion (e.g., composing the "Union Jack" figure from a series of small triangles). Quite often these errors of approach or assembly of drawings would be missed if the drawing process were not observed and only the completed figure inspected.

Common distortions of the Gesell drawings are shown under each of the drawings in Figure 3-1 and include the following:

1. Circle—at an approximate 30 month level, a child will imitate circular motions, but will not stop with satisfactory completion of a circle.
2. Intersecting lines—at an approximate 27 month level a child will imitate horizontal and vertical strokes. The most common distortion in copying intersecting lines is shown in Figure 3-1.
3. Square—the most common distortion of a square includes partial replication of a square with the remainder of the figure completed with a circular motion as shown in Figure 3-1. This distorted figure represents a synthesis of the circle and square and is at an approximate 3.5 year level.
4. Triangle—the most common distortion of the triangle includes a right angle with the remainder of the figure completed with a sloping line. The resultant drawing looks more like a right triangle.
5. "Union Jack"—the most common distortion is drawing the figure in a fragmented fashion (as a series of pie slices or with spokes radiating out from a central focus). Another common distortion is shown in Figure 3-1.
6. Vertical diamond—the most common distortion is drawing the figure as a square tipped on its side rather than as a diamond.
7. Maltese Cross—distortions include unequal arm heights and widths.
8. Cylinder—this is the first figure in the series that is three-dimensional. The most common distortion of the figure is a drawing with a circular top or flat bottom, missing the concept that the figure has depth into the page.
9. Opaque three-dimensional cube—again this is a three-dimensional figure, and the most common distortion is to draw it as a series of flat squares or with poor perspective. Quite often, when one observes a child who has extreme difficulty in copying this last figure, comparable difficulty may be observed in the parent's replication of this same figure. If this process can be conducted in a tactful fashion, it may help the parents bet-

ter understand their child's visual perceptual difficulties. The parents may have learned to rationalize their own perceptual difficulties by defenses of the type, "I never liked art." In effect, what they may well share with their child is an unrecognized visual perceptual deficit.

Assessment of Visual Perceptual Development-Block Performance

Earlier in this chapter, the use of one-inch cubes was discussed in the assessment of visual perceptual abilities for preschool children. Two of the block constructions presented in Table 3-4 (staircase assemblies f and g) may be useful for assessing visual problem solving for early school-age (5 to 7 years) children.

The relationships among visual perceptual deficits, the type of learning disabilities encountered, and the most effective modes of remediation are quite unclear. It is still taken on faith that children with visual perceptual deficits will have more substantial difficulties with letter and shape recognition and will have more difficulty perceiving whole words visually as gestalts. Intuitively it seems reasonable to suppose that a careful evaluation of a child's strengths and weaknesses would be useful in remediation planning, although sadly this has not been a very straightforward process.

Short-Term Memory Assessment

Short-term memory is tested with digits forward, digits reversed, and sentence memory (Table 3-6). Qualitative deviance may be noted when a child remembers the digits, but does not get them in the correct order (sequential memory deficit rather than a rote auditory memory deficit). Additionally, the child with ADHD frequently exhibits an inconsistent performance with digit recall, doing somewhat better when attention is focused carefully and distractions minimized. The child with ADHD also may exhibit better ability to reverse digits than to perform them forward.

Handedness, Laterality, and Dominance

Numerous authors have observed developmentally inappropriate right-left confusion, failure to establish hand preference at an appropriate age, and problems with laterality (child's awareness of the two sides of his body and ability to identify them as left and right) in dyslexic children. Tests of right-left discrimination and laterality are included in Table 3-7.

TABLE 3-6
Auditory Memory

Digits Forward—Digits spaced approximately 1 second apart

2.5	yr	47 _____	63 _____	58 _____
3	yr	641 _____	352 _____	837 _____
4.5	yr	4729 _____	3852 _____	7261 _____
7	yr	31589 _____	48372 _____	96183 _____
10	yr	473859 _____	429746 _____	728394 _____
Adult		72594836 _____	47153962 _____	41935826 _____

Digits Reversed

7	yr	295 _____	816 _____	473 _____
9	yr	8526 _____	4937 _____	3629 _____
12	yr	81379 _____	69582 _____	52618 _____
Adult		471952 _____	583694 _____	752618 _____

Sentences—Read at a normal rate

4 yr   We are going to buy some candy for mother.
Jack likes to feed the little puppies in the barn.

5 yr   Jane wants to build a big castle in her playhouse.
Tom has lots of fun playing ball with his sister.

8 yr   Fred asked his father to take him to see the clowns in the circus.
Billy made a beautiful boat out of wood with his sharp knife.

11 yr   At the summer camp the children get up early in the morning and go swimming.
Yesterday we went for a ride in our car along the road that crosses the bridge.

13 yr   The airplane made a careful landing in the space which had been prepared for it.
Tom Brown's dog ran quickly down the road with a huge bone in his mouth.

Adult   The red headed woodpecker made a terrible fuss as they tried to drive the young away from the nest.
The early settlers had little idea of the great changes that were to take place in this country.

TABLE 3-7
Left-Right Discrimination Testing

Show me your *left* hand Show me your *right* eye	4.5 yr
Put your *left* hand on your *left* eye Put your *right* hand on your *right* ear	4.5 yr
Put your *left* hand on your *right* eye Put your *right* hand on your *left* ear	5.5 yr
Touch my *right* hand Touch my *left* knee	7.5 yr
Put your *left* hand on my *right* hand Put your *right* hand on my *left* knee	7.5 yr
Put your *left* hand on my *left* knee Put your *right* hand on my *right* hand	7.5 yr

There is, however, no conclusive evidence to support the proposition that these developmental problems are related to a failure to establish asymmetrical functions of the two brain hemispheres. Furthermore, neither mixed dominance (e.g., preference for the right hand but the left eye) nor left-handedness per se seem to be related to learning disabilities in children.

There are several "red flags" of underlying significant pathology related to the issue of handedness with preschool children:

1. Establishment of handedness below 1 year of age is an abnormal finding, and until proven otherwise should be construed as equivalent to a hemiparesis (relative motor disability on one side of the body).
2. Failure to develop hand preference by 2 years of age should be considered equally suspect.

Soft Neurological Signs

The classical neurological examination looks at what are termed *hard neurological signs*, that is, neurological findings that either are present or absent and do not appear to be modified by maturation of the child's nervous system. In this context, the presence or absence of neurological findings is used to identify the presence of and permit localization of pathology in the nervous system. In the child's developing nervous system, however, things are not so simple. The physician performing a neurological examination with a child's developing nervous system is faced with neurological findings that are on a developmental continuum, that is, they appear and disappear with development and maturation of the nervous system. Pathology here does not equate simply with the presence or absence of physical findings, but rather will depend on the extent of their presence and the timing of their appearance and disappearance. This fact has led to a great deal of confusion in interpreting the significance of these *soft neurological signs*. It has been demonstrated that, despite some variability on serial examination, soft signs can have a reasonably high interexaminer reliability and their presence may correlate significantly with learning disabilities.

`Between one-third and one-half of children with learning problems demonstrate significant soft neurological signs. Mirror movements and synkinesias (associated movements) represent the most commonly encountered soft neurological signs. Mirror movements are associated movements of the opposite extremity that arise when a specific request is made for isolated movements of one of the extremities. Synkinesias represent an overflow or overshooting of muscle movements into other surrounding muscle groups when a request is made for performance with an isolated muscle group. Both mirror movements and synkinesias are commonly encountered in children with learning disabilities, but their presence is not pathognomonic.

CONCLUSION

The physician, because of early and ongoing contact with the child, is in an opportune position to identify early delays that may portend subsequent learning difficulties. This chapter has described how the physician, through an expanded neurodevelopmental history and neurodevelopmental examination, can make an individual contribution in this early identification process. With older children, and with further progression of learning disabilities, the physician can be a valuable participant in the interdisciplinary diagnostic and therapeutic process. The role of the physician in the interdisciplinary process will be discussed in subsequent chapters.

CHAPTER 4

Psychological Evaluation

Elizabeth H. Aylward

As mentioned previously, the diagnosis of learning disabilities is based on evidence of a discrepancy between the child's cognitive abilities and academic achievement, when other handicapping conditions (e.g., sensory impairment, mental retardation, social and emotional disturbance) or environmental influences (e.g., cultural differences, insufficient or inappropriate instruction, psychogenic factors) have been ruled out as primary reasons for the discrepancy. The psychologist plays an important role in making the diagnosis by providing information regarding the child's cognitive functioning, as well as by providing information that helps rule out other conditions, and information that helps to explain the nature of the disabilities.

HISTORY TAKING

Like the physician, the psychologist is in an excellent position to gather important information from the parents that may assist in understanding the child's school difficulties. Some of the questions will necessarily overlap with those included in the physician's interview and in the special educator's information-gathering process. It is not a waste of time to have questions repeated by various professionals, as it will provide each professional with a clearer understanding of the parents' perception of the problems. Furthermore, parents are bound to share different bits and pieces of the puzzle with different professionals, even if the questions asked are identical. This will allow for a clearer view of the "big picture" when the team gets together to share information.

The psychologist will want to gather information from the parents either before or after testing the child. She may want to ask about the child's school history, if this information is not already available from the special educator's report. Included in the school history will be information regarding number of years at the current school, previous schools attended and years of attendance, preschools attended and years of attendance, regularity of attendance, reasons for excessive absences, problems noted by teachers throughout the grades, special education services provided in previous years, any repetitions of grades or specific courses, types of remedial efforts that have been attempted, and the outcome of these efforts. The psychologist will want to ask parents about their perceptions of current behavior problems at school and perceptions of strengths and weaknesses in the various subject areas. The psychologist will also want to explore issues that relate to the child's success and satisfaction with school, including ability to interact with peers (both at home and at school), involvement in extracurricular activities, and self-concept.

In order to determine if problems observed in school are unique to the school situation or more pervasive, the psychologist should ask about behavior problems at home (e.g., excessive activity level, tantrums, inability to listen to and follow instructions, lying, stealing, refusal to do what is asked). The psychologist should ask about homework: how much is assigned (in the parents' estimation), how long it actually takes the child to complete the work, whether parental supervision is required, and particular problems with completion of homework (e.g., procrastination, whining, distractibility, need for assistance). The child's ability to carry out other responsibilities (e.g., regular daily chores) should also be discussed.

The psychologist should question the parent regarding the presence of symptoms of depression or other emotional disturbance in the child (e.g., unusual fears, sleeping problems, eating problems, mood swings, difficulty separating from parents). The psychologist may want to ask questions regarding any learning, emotional, or behavior problems in other family members. Finally, the psychologist should ask whether the child is currently taking any medication which might interfere with testing and, if so, whether the medication was administered on the day of psychological testing.

An interview form that the psychologist might want to use with parents is included in Appendix A. Of course, the psychologist will want to modify the form to suit his individual needs.

PSYCHOLOGICAL TESTING

The basis for a diagnosis of learning disabilities is performance on individually administered tests of intelligence and academic achievement. As explained previously, a learning disability exists when academic achievement in one or more areas is significantly lower than the level that would be predicted from the child's cognitive profile, assuming that other conditions (e.g., emotional disturbance, excessive school absences, vision or hearing problems, inappropriate educational techniques) are not present. It is clear, then, that accurate assessments of both academic achievement and intellectual abilities are essential for accurate diagnosis. The psychologist is generally responsible for the assessment of intellectual abilities, whereas the educator is responsible for assessment of academic achievement.

Test Selection

Because the accurate assessment of intelligence is essential to the diagnosis of learning disabilities, it is imperative that the psychologist select a valid and reliable instrument that measures the child's intellectual abilities in such a way that is not biased by the child's lack of academic achievement. There is, of course, no single, correct definition of "intelligence." Therefore, there is no single, correct way of measuring this concept. The examiner must be aware of the types of cognitive abilities tapped by the various intelligence tests in order to select the test(s) that will provide the most valid results for his or her population of students.

Individually Administered IQ Tests

Although most school systems now have adopted programs of testing at regular intervals throughout the elementary and secondary school years, these tests are typically administered to students in large groups (20 or more students). Although these tests provide fairly accurate evaluations of academic skills (and sometimes overall intellectual ability) for many students, they are especially inappropriate for children suspected of having learning disabilities. First, many children with learning disabilities have concomitant attention deficits, and they are at particular disadvantage in a group testing situation, especially if the tests are administered with a time limit. A group testing situation is a perfect environment for daydreaming and other off-task behaviors for the child with attention deficit disorder. Second, most group tests require the student to read the items himself. Although poor reading abilities will be more or less accurately reflected in reading subtest scores on group tests, they will provide a serious confounding variable in the measurement of other academic abilities (e.g., social studies, applied math, study skills) and overall cognitive abilities. Third, group testing does not provide the examiner with an opportunity to closely observe many of the behaviors that interfere with testing and similarly interfere with classroom learning (e.g., limited attention span, impulsivity, excessive frustration). For these reasons, individual testing is essential for correct diagnosis of learning disabilities.

Selection of a Test of Intellectual Functioning

In making a diagnosis of learning disabilities the minimum information necessary is an accurate assessment of intelligence (often in the form of an "IQ" score) and an accurate assessment of academic achievement in one or more areas. Although many tests on the market claim to provide an "IQ" or other score reflecting overall cognitive ability, few are appropriate in making the diagnosis of learning disabilities.

In a 1984 report of the United States Department of Education, Special Education Programs Work Group on Management Issues in the Assessment of Learning Disabilities (Reynolds, 1984), eleven considerations were presented for selection of instruments used in the diagnosis of learning disabilities. These are presented in Table 4-1. Basically, these standards require tests used for the diagnosis of learning disabilities to meet generally accepted criteria for reliability (i.e., ability of a test to consistently measure what it measures) and validity (i.e., ability of a test to actually measure what it purports to measure). Furthermore, the test norms must be based on a sufficiently large sample that reflects the demographic characteristics of the national population. The test norms should allow the examiner to compare the child with other children of the same age. The degree to which different ethnic and cultural populations perform differently on the test should have been studied and reported. The test of cognitive abilities should measure "general" intelligence. Another primary consideration is the need for the test of cognitive ability and the test of academic achievement to be normed on the same or similar populations.

In addition to these important criteria, it is desirable to use an intelligence test that allows the examiner to observe the child over a range of response modes (e.g., single-word responses, elaborated oral responses, paper-and-pencil tasks, manipulation of materials, identification by pointing, imitation of the examiner, timed and untimed responses). The test should also tap various aspects of intelligence.

TABLE 4-1
Essential Characteristics of Tests Used in Making the Diagnosis of Learning Disabilities

1. Tests should meet all requirements stated for assessment devices in the rules and regulations implementing Public Law 94-142.

2. Normative data should meet contemporary standards of practice and be provided for a sufficiently large, nationally stratified random sample of children.

3. Standardization samples for tests whose scores are being compared must be the same or highly comparable.

4. For the purpose of arriving at a diagnosis, individually administered tests should be used.

5. In the measurement of aptitude, an individually administered test of general intellectual ability should be used.

6. Age-based standard scores should be used for all measures and all should be scaled to a common metric.

7. The measures employed should demonstrate a high level of reliability and have appropriate studies for this determination in the technical manual accompanying the test.

8. The validity coefficient r_{xy}, representing the relationship between the measures of aptitude and achievement, should be based on an appropriate sample.

9. Validity of test score interpretations should be clearly established.

10. Special technical considerations should be addressed when using performance-based measures of achievement (e.g., writing skill).

11. Bias studies on the instruments in use should have been conducted and reported.

Adapted from Reynolds, C. (1984–1985). Critical measurement issues in learning disabilities. *Journal of Special Education, 18*(4), 451–476.

WISC-R, Stanford-Binet, and K-ABC

Three intelligence tests that generally meet the technical criteria described (validity, reliability, adequate norming samples) and that are most commonly used are the Wechsler Intelligence Scale for Children-Revised (WISC-R), the Stanford-Binet (Fourth Edition; hereafter, "Stanford-Binet" refers to the Fourth Edition), and the Kaufman Assessment Battery for Children (K-ABC). (See Aylward, 1991, for a description of each of these tests.) There is, of course, much debate regarding the nature of intelligence and the types of tasks that should be used to measure intelligence. The K-ABC, Stanford-Binet, and WISC-R differ considerably in their approach to defining and measuring intelligence. None of these tests can be considered "right" or "wrong" in their approach. The examiner will have to consider the nature of the individual tasks used within each of these tests of intelligence to determine which is the best choice for each child he or she diagnoses.

The two major aspects of intelligence measured by the WISC-R are verbal (language) and nonverbal (primarily visual-spatial) skills. The Stanford-Binet is designed to measure "crystallized abilities" (verbal reasoning and quantitative reasoning), "fluid-analytic abilities" (abstract/visual reasoning), and short-term memory. The K-ABC has been designed to measure "simultaneous" and "sequential" mental processing. On tasks measuring Sequential Mental Processing, stimuli are manipulated in serial order to solve problems; on tasks measuring Simultaneous Mental Processing, stimuli are integrated in a holistic, gestalt, or parallel fashion to solve problems. Intelligence, as measured by the K-ABC, is considered to be "an individual's style of solving problems and processing information" (Kaufman & Kaufman, 1983, p. 2). The K-ABC attempts to "minimize the role of language and acquired facts and skills" (Kaufman, 1983, p. 206). Although many of the subtests on the WISC-R and Stanford-Binet are similar to K-ABC subtests in measuring problem-solving and information-processing styles, the WISC-R and Stanford-Binet also include other subtests that definitely rely on learned material for good performance. The type of learning required on these subtests is, however, the type that is generally picked up in day-to-day living (e.g., vocabulary, understanding of social situations, general information), rather than that which relies on direct school learning.

Because the K-ABC and the Stanford-Binet are newer than the WISC-R, they are less widely used, and their advantages and disadvantages are less widely understood. It is recommended that the psychologist on the interdisciplinary team be familiar with all three of these intelligence tests. He or she will find it more appropriate to use one or the other in various situations. Although it is impossible to identify the K-ABC, Stanford-Binet, or WISC-R as the "best" test for measuring intelligence as part of the diagnostic process, there are certain considerations that the psychologist should consider in each individual case:

1. One of the major advantages of using the K-ABC instead of the WISC-R or Stanford-Binet is the availability of the K-ABC Achievement subtests, which were normed on the same sample as the K-ABC Mental Processing subtests. This allows the examiner to confidently compare results of the intelligence measure and the academic achieve-

ment measures, which is essential in making the diagnosis of learning disabilities. Unfortunately, however, many examiners think the K-ABC Achievement subtests do not adequately test several important academic skills (e.g., spelling, application of phonics skills, written calculations) that commonly are measured by achievement tests.

2. The K-ABC, unlike the WISC-R, includes in its norming sample exceptional children (e.g., children who are learning-disabled, mentally retarded, gifted) in the same proportion as occurs in the national population. The Stanford-Binet norming sample included some exceptional students, but it is not clear what types and what proportions of exceptional students were involved. Inclusion of exceptional students in the norming sample increases validity of the scores for the individual exceptional student.

3. Because the K-ABC and Stanford-Binet are newer tests than the WISC-R, the children in their standardization samples probably are more similar to children currently being evaluated than the children in the WISC-R standardization sample, thus increasing the chance for validity. An important point to be noted in the use of tests for diagnosing learning disabilities is the necessity for a high degree of comparability of standardization samples for tests whose scores are being compared. That is, when the scores from two tests (e.g., an intelligence test and an achievement test) are to be compared, the samples on which those two tests were normed should be highly similar. The most widely used tests of academic achievement have been standardized within the past 10 years. Because the WISC-R was normed in the early 1970s, its standardization sample may be less similar to the standardization samples used in norming the widely used tests of academic achievement than are the K-ABC's and Stanford-Binet's standardization samples. Thus, comparisons between scores from a test of intelligence and scores from tests of academic achievement may be more valid if the K-ABC or Stanford-Binet is used. Renorming of the WISC-R is, however, currently underway, so concern about the age of the norms will no longer be a consideration with the arrival of the WISC-III.

4. Racial and ethnic differences are less pronounced on the K-ABC, and perhaps the Stanford-Binet, than on the WISC-R. For example, Kaufman (1983) reports a 7-point average difference between the scores of black children and white children on the K-ABC, whereas an average difference of 16 points is reported for the WISC-R (Kaufman & Doppelt, 1976). A similar trend is reported for the differences between scores of Hispanic and white children. The developers of the Stanford-Binet had a large staff representing various minority groups review all of the test items for the possibility of racial, ethnic, or gender bias. This procedure resulted in some items being revised or dropped.

However, the test developers do not provide information regarding differences in scores among various racial or ethnic groups or sexes.

5. All K-ABC Mental Processing subtests include teaching or training items. These allow the examiner to use various means to make certain that the child understands the task. Although the WISC-R and Stanford-Binet provide sample items for most subtests (which allow the examiner to correct mistakes, using a clearly prescribed protocol), these sample items do not always ensure that the child understands what is expected. This situation, of course, is a more serious problem with younger or less intelligent children. The K-ABC teaching items allow the examiner to be more certain that a low score reflects a true weakness in a skill area rather than an inability to understand directions.

6. The K-ABC provides a Nonverbal Scale, made up of subtests that can be administered in pantomime and responded to motorically. This scale is designed for children who are hearing impaired, who have serious speech or language disorders, or who use English as a second language. Although many of the WISC-R Performance subtests require no verbal response, it might be difficult to communicate the instructions for the task to a child with hearing impairment. Furthermore, this situation definitely would be considered "nonstandard" procedure for administration of the WISC-R subtests, thus invalidating norms. The Stanford-Binet suggests alternate batteries that can be given to students with limited English proficiency or hearing deficits, but special norms for these batteries are not provided.

7. The K-ABC provides a variety of supplementary norms, including sociocultural norms (based on a cross-tabulation by race and by parental education). Thus, children can, when desired, be compared with peers from similar sociocultural backgrounds.

8. The K-ABC provides specific strategies for teaching reading, math, and spelling, based on the child's profile of strengths and weaknesses on the Simultaneous versus Sequential Mental Processing tasks. (The effectiveness of these strategies, however, has not been proven yet.)

9. Although the K-ABC intentionally omitted tasks that require extensive verbal expression, it cannot be denied that this is an ability that contributes greatly to school success. The examiner may want information comparing verbal and nonverbal skills, which can be obtained much more directly and thoroughly from the WISC-R, and to a lesser extent from the Stanford-Binet, than from the K-ABC.

10. Just as the K-ABC may be useful for testing children who are hearing impaired or who have serious speech or language disorders, the WISC-R Verbal subtests may be useful for assessing cognitive abilities of children who are visually impaired. These children would be seriously disadvantaged on the K-ABC tests. The Stanford-Binet suggests alterna-

tive batteries for children who are blind or visually impaired. None of these tests provide special norms for children who are visually impaired.

11. The WISC-R and Stanford-Binet allow the examiner to observe the child over a greater range of response modes than the K-ABC. Manipulation of objects, paper-and-pencil skills, single-word responses, elaborated oral responses, identification by pointing, and imitation of the examiner are all required by the various WISC-R and Stanford-Binet tasks. Although individual scores are not obtained for each of these response modes, the experienced examiner can use his or her observation to formulate some fairly sophisticated hypotheses regarding certain factors that will interfere with the child's learning. Most of the responses on the K-ABC require identification by pointing, although a few require single word responses, manipulation of objects, or imitation of the examiner.

12. The WISC-R and Stanford-Binet employ more manipulative materials than the K-ABC. Although this makes administration of the WISC-R and Stanford-Binet somewhat more cumbersome, it may be more effective in keeping the child's attention (especially at younger ages).

13. Because of its "adaptive-testing" procedure, the Stanford Binet is definitely the most difficult of the three tests to learn to administer. The WISC-R generally is considered to be a more difficult test to learn to administer than the K-ABC. Also, because scoring on several of the WISC-R and Stanford-Binet subtests is somewhat subjective, examiners with less testing experience may have more difficulty scoring these tests as accurately as the K-ABC.

14. The three tests are designed to cover different age ranges, with the WISC-R covering ages 6 to 16, the K-ABC covering ages 2 years 6 months to 12 years 6 months, and the Stanford-Binet covering ages 2 through adult. Younger children or those with significant delays often are unable to reach basal level on several of the Stanford-Binet subtests. For very young children, the K-ABC would be an appropriate test to use, although examiners might wish to supplement it with some measure of verbal ability. The Wechsler Preschool and Primary Scale of Intelligence-Revised (WPPSI-R), which provides norms for children ages 3 through 7 years, also is an excellent test for preschool children. For individuals above age 16, the Wechsler Adult Intelligence Scale-Revised (WAIS-R) should be considered, as the norms for older individuals on the Stanford-Binet only go through age 23 years 11 months and are based on a large single sample for individuals between 18 and 24.

15. Because the WISC-R has been available much longer, it is better known and better understood by most professionals than the two newer tests. The psychologist who chooses to use the K-ABC or Stan-

ford-Binet probably will have to spend more time explaining the scales and their meaning. This consideration will, of course, become less valid if and when the K-ABC and Stanford-Binet become more widely used.

The Woodcock-Johnson Psychoeducational Battery-Revised

The Woodcock-Johnson Psychoeducational Battery-Revised (WJ-R) consists of two sections: Tests of Cognitive Ability and Tests of Achievement. The Tests of Cognitive Ability (WJ-R COG) sometimes are used as a measure of intellectual functioning for the diagnosis of learning disabilities. Although there are some advantages to using the WJ-R COG as a measure of intelligence (e.g., excellent technical qualities, ease of administration, availability of the companion set of academic achievement tests), the disadvantages prevent it from being the test of choice for the purpose of diagnosing learning disabilities.

The primary complaint regarding the original Woodcock-Johnson Psychoeducational Battery (published in 1977) concerned the unusual assortment of cognitive tasks chosen to represent the construct of intelligence. In fact, the developers of the original version did not even consider the test to be an intelligence test per se. Unlike its predecessor, the WJ-R COG clearly is based on a model of intelligence (the Horn-Cattell theory), and is designed to measure seven of the broad intellectual abilities defined by this theory. Nevertheless, the seven tests selected for the Standard Battery are a somewhat unusual representation of overall cognitive functioning, appearing to be rather heavily weighted toward tasks that are at a fairly low level of cognitive complexity (e.g., rote memory, psychomotor speed). For this reason, the WJ-R COG is not recommended as a test of intelligence for the evaluation of learning disabilities.

Appropriate Tests of Intelligence for Preschool Children

As discussed in Chapter 2, early identification of children with learning disabilities is desirable, as emphasized under P. L. 99-457. As part of this early identification procedure, it is essential for the psychologist to obtain a measure of overall cognitive function. The K-ABC and Stanford Binet can provide measures of cognitive abilities for children as young as 2 years 6 months. As noted earlier, the WISC-R is designed for children who are at least 6 years old. The Wechsler Preschool and Primary Scale of Intelligence-Revised (WPPSI-R) is similar to the WISC-R and is designed for children between the ages of 3 and 7 years. The WPPSI-R is described fully by Aylward (1991).

Appropriate Tests of Intelligence for Older Children

The K-ABC cannot be used with children over 12 years 6 months, and the WISC-R cannot be used with children over 16 years 11 months. The Wechsler Adult Intelligence Scale-Revised (WAIS-R) is similar to the WISC-R and WPPSI-R in content, and is designed for individuals who are 16 years or older. It contains the same six Verbal subtests as the WISC-R; the Mazes subtest is omitted from the Performance subtests. Of course, items are more difficult.

Inappropriate Tests of Intelligence for the Diagnosis of Learning Disabilities

As mentioned previously, it is important that the intelligence test selected for use in making the diagnosis of learning disabilities be individually administered, have adequate validity and reliability, include tasks that tap a variety of aspects of intelligence, and provide the examiner an opportunity to observe the student over a range of response modes. There are several commonly used "intelligence" tests that do not meet these criteria and are, therefore, inappropriate for making the diagnosis of learning disabilities. Among this group of inappropriate, but commonly used tests, is the Slosson Intelligence Test (SIT), which is inappropriate because it is inadequately normed on an unrepresentative sample and contains too few items at each age level. The Peabody Picture Vocabulary Test-Revised (PPVT-R), the Full Range Picture Vocabulary Test, and the Quick Test are inappropriate because they measure only limited aspects of receptive vocabulary skills. The Standard Progressive Matrices test is equally inappropriate for making the diagnosis of learning disabilities because it measures only limited aspects of visual-spatial reasoning. As described previously, the diagnosis of learning disabilities requires scores based on individually administered tests that allow the examiner to monitor closely the child's test behavior and to ensure maximum attention. For this reason, group administered tests of intelligence (e.g., the Otis-Lennon Mental Ability Test, California Test of Mental Maturity) are inappropriate.

Although some of these "inappropriate" tests may be useful as screening tools for identifying children with possible learning disabilities, they certainly should not be used as the measure of intelligence for making a final diagnosis. Similarly, a child who does not show a significant discrepancy between academic achievement and intellectual ability, as measured by one of these tests, should not be assumed to be free of learning disabilities if other indications of the disorder are observed.

Test Administration

Appropriate Test Conditions

As outlined in any introductory text of assessment or any manual for an individually administered test, a proper test environment is essential for accurate assessment. This situation is especially true for the child with learning disabilities who is often easily distracted. The testing room must, of course, be quiet, free from excessive visual distractions, properly ventilated, of comfortable temperature, and equipped with furniture that allows the child to be seated comfortably at a table or desk. Several of the tests most useful in diagnosing learning disabilities will not provide reliable results if such conditions are not maintained.

If possible, the child should be tested in the morning when he is well-rested and alert. Tests should be administered in sessions no longer than two hours (or shorter for younger children). If tests must be administered in one session, the student should be allowed a short break in the middle of the session.

The examiner should make a special attempt to build rapport with the child being evaluated for possible learning disabilities. Many of these children, after years of poor academic achievement, have poor self-esteem, are easily frustrated, poorly motivated, or overly anxious. To obtain an accurate assessment of the student's abilities, the examiner must take into account these emotional interferences and must attempt to overcome them.

Behaviors to be Observed During Intelligence Testing

The psychologist administering the test of cognitive abilities should include in his or her report a section on behavioral observations of the child in the testing situation. Some of the behaviors that should be addressed in this section of the report are discussed in the next paragraphs. If these behavioral observations are not included in the report, the psychologist should be contacted and questioned directly about the following:

Distractibility
- ☐ Did the child have difficulty paying attention and staying on task? Did the child appear to be day dreaming, or off in his or her own world?
- ☐ Did the child often ask to have items repeated?
- ☐ Did the child often comment about or seem attuned to unavoidable visual or auditory distractions (e.g., the squeaking of a chair, the examiner's clothing)?

PSYCHOLOGICAL EVALUATION

☐ Did the child make irrelevant comments or attempt to relate personal experiences that were brought to mind by the various test stimuli? Did the child often talk to him- or herself, especially on tasks that required manipulation of materials rather than a verbal response?

☐ Did he seem to "lose track" of the task presented? For example, on the "digits reversed" section of the WISC-R Digit Span subtest, did the child begin to repeat digits forward after several successful trials of repeating digits in reversed order? On the WISC-R Coding subtest did the child stop in the middle of the test, seeming to have forgotten instructions to work as quickly as possible? Did the child frequently lose his or her place on the Coding subtest?

Restlessness, Fidgetiness

☐ Did the child have difficulty staying seated, especially on the subtests that did not require manipulation of materials?

☐ Did restlessness increase as testing proceeded or stay at a constant level?

☐ Did the child engage in excessive purposeless movement (e.g., squirming, tapping fingers, swinging feet, kicking the table leg)? Were the child's hands overly "busy" (e.g., repetitively rolling his hands in his shirt tail, twirling his pencil, picking at himself)?

☐ Did the child chew on his or her pencil, shirt collar, cuffs, or other objects?

Rushed, Careless, Impulsive Approach

☐ Did the child appear to give the first answer that came to mind?

☐ Did the child attempt to begin tasks before instructions were complete?

☐ Did the child attempt to turn pages before adequately attending to the material on the current page?

☐ Did the child grab for materials before the examiner was ready to present them?

☐ Did the child appear totally oblivious to obviously incorrect responses?

☐ Did the child noticeably increase his or her speed of responding when he or she was aware that performance was being timed? Did this result in careless errors?

Slow, Obsessive Approach

☐ Did the child take excessive time before responding?

☐ Did the child meticulously check and recheck work, resulting in penalties for slow performance?

- [ ] Were the child's verbal responses more complete than necessary (especially on vocabulary and comprehension subtests)?
- [ ] Did the child often come up with correct responses *after* time was called?
- [ ] Did the child spend excessive time "planning" before responding (especially on WISC-R Mazes or K-ABC Photo Series)?
- [ ] Were tasks done with excessive precision (e.g., were blocks on the WISC-R Block Design or triangles on the K-ABC Triangles subtests lined up exactly, lines drawn extremely neatly or overworked on Stanford-Binet Copying)?

Anxiety
- [ ] Did the child have difficulty separating from his or her parent or teacher?
- [ ] Did the child appear nervous? Did this subside or increase as testing proceeded? Did it diminish with positive reinforcement and reassurance?
- [ ] Did anxiety appear to increase when tasks were timed?
- [ ] Was more anxiety observed on certain types of tasks (e.g., those requiring a verbal response, those that were timed) than on other types of tasks?

Confidence
- [ ] Did the child ask often if his or her responses were correct?
- [ ] Was the child reluctant to guess at an item he or she did not know?
- [ ] Could the child be encouraged to take a guess, and, if so, were guesses often correct?
- [ ] Did the child start to give answers and then change his or her mind and refuse to respond?
- [ ] Did the child qualify many responses (e.g., by saying, "I don't know, but . . ." or "This is just a guess.")?
- [ ] Did the child often comment on the difficulty of items (e.g., "These are so easy" or "I'll never get this one.")? Were these assessments of difficulty congruent with the child's performance?
- [ ] Did the child often say "I can't" or "I don't know" without putting forth good effort?
- [ ] Did the child often ask for assistance on items or look to the examiner for reassurance that he was "on the right track"?

Frustration—Perseverance
- [ ] Did the child often stop working on a task before time was called, claiming an item was too difficult? Could he or she be

PSYCHOLOGICAL EVALUATION

encouraged to continue and, if so, was he or she able to successfully complete the item?
- [ ] If unable to succeed on an item within the time limit, did the child request "just a little longer" to complete the task?
- [ ] Did the child ever scatter materials in frustration?
- [ ] Did the child act disgusted with him- or herself or make disparaging comments when he or she could not succeed on an item?
- [ ] Did the child ever ask to complete remaining items after failing the prescribed number of items for discontinuing the testing?

Distortions in Spatial Orientation
- [ ] Did the child have many rotations on WISC-R Block Design, Stanford-Binet Pattern Analysis, or K-ABC Triangles?
- [ ] Did the child work from right to left when sequencing WISC-R Picture Arrangement cards or completing the WISC-R Coding task?

Pencil Grasp
- [ ] Did the child exhibit an immature or awkward pencil grasp on the WISC-R Coding and Mazes subtests or on the Stanford-Binet Copying subtest?

Avoidance Behavior
- [ ] Did the child ask for excessive breaks (e.g., for bathroom visits, drinks)?
- [ ] Did the child complain of stomach aches or other ailments in an apparent attempt to discontinue the session?
- [ ] Did the child complain of being tired?
- [ ] Did the child often ask how much longer the testing would last?
- [ ] Did the child complain about the testing?

Hearing and Vision
- [ ] Were there any indications that the child had difficulty seeing materials or hearing questions (e.g., squinting, holding materials close to his or her face, often saying "huh?" or asking to have questions repeated)?

Speech and Language
- [ ] Did the child often ask to have verbal items repeated?
- [ ] Was the child slow to begin giving verbal responses?
- [ ] Did the child often appear to not understand verbal directions, but "catch on" quickly after a few demonstration items?

☐ Did the child have "word finding" problems. For example, did the child often refer to objects on the WISC-R Picture Completion subtest as "those things" or "what-cha-ma-call-its"? Did he or she often give a long verbal explanation to describe something for which more concise terminology would have been more appropriate?
☐ Were verbal responses extremely limited? Did the child resist your encouragement to elaborate on verbal responses?
☐ Did the child give totally inappropriate responses to verbal questions and then, upon repetition of the question, provide an accurate response?
☐ Did the child give responses which related only to a portion of the question?
☐ Did the child have any observable speech impediments (e.g., stuttering, lisping, poor articulation)? Did they interfere with testing?

Personality Characteristics
☐ Was the child friendly, pleasant, well-mannered, cooperative?
☐ Did the child appear well-motivated?
☐ Did the child appear to enjoy the testing and the individual attention of the examiner?
☐ Did the child offer spontaneous conversation?
☐ Did the child make eye-contact with the examiner?
☐ Did the child appear to take pride in his successes? Did he or she respond to praise?
☐ Did the child respond to the examiner's attempts to build rapport?
☐ Was the child overly affectionate with the examiner?

Health
☐ Was the child on any type of medication that might have affected performance (e.g., Ritalin, antihistamines)?
☐ Were there any other health conditions that might have affected performance?

Although this list of behavioral observations may seem quite lengthy and detailed, it is important that each area be considered. The psychologist may even want to make a checklist to use during testing to facilitate reporting of these characteristics. Some of the child's major difficulties may be reflected more in these behavioral traits than in any test score. Recommendations for remediation of school difficulties certainly will need to take these traits into account.

Test Interpretation

WISC-R VIQ-PIQ Discrepancy and Subtest Scatter

Many attempts have been made to identify "the learning disability profile" of subtest scores on the WISC-R. Despite the fact that no consistent profile has been found, some psychologists and educators may attempt to make a diagnosis of learning disabilities based on the WISC-R profile alone. This approach is not appropriate. Most commonly, these inappropriate diagnoses are based on an extreme amount of subtest scatter or on a significant discrepancy between VIQ and PIQ. Although students with learning disabilities often show great subtest scatter (i.e., differences in performance among the various subtests) and VIQ-PIQ discrepancies, there are many children without learning disabilities who also show these "abnormal" patterns, and there are many students with learning disabilities who do not show these patterns.

Compounding the problem, many professionals who work primarily with children exhibiting school difficulties are unaware of the amount of subtest scatter and VIQ-PIQ discrepancy found in the profile of the "normal" child. In examining the standardization data for the WISC-R, Kaufman (1976b) discovered that the average VIQ-PIQ discrepancy (regardless of direction) was 9.7 points. The values for determining whether a particular VIQ-PIQ discrepancy is "real" (i.e., not due to chance) are 9 points ($p < 0.15$ level), 12 ($p < 0.05$ level), and 15 points ($p < 0.01$ level). Kaufman considers a VIQ-PIQ discrepancy of 12 points or more (regardless or direction) worthy of explanation. It is important to note, however, that a discrepancy of this size is, by no means "abnormal," as it is observed in approximately 34 percent of the normal population. Table 4-2 reports the percentage of normal children who have VIQ-PIQ discrepancies of various magnitudes.

Substantial scatter among the twelve WISC-R subtests also is not unusual. Two-thirds of children have scaled score ranges (the difference between the highest and lowest subtest score) of 7 + 2 points. An "abnormal" amount of scatter (that which occurs in less than 15 percent of normal children) is present when there is a spread of 8 points or more between the highest and lowest of the six Verbal subtest scores, and when there is a spread of 9 points or more between the highest and lowest of the six Performance subtest scores (based on a study by Kaufman, 1976a, which examined WISC-R profiles of 2,200 normal children). (See Table 4-3.)

Because VIQ-PIQ discrepancies and the amount of subtest scatter in normal populations is larger than many examiners would suspect, and because these intra-test comparisons cannot accurately identify

TABLE 4-2
Percentage of Nondisabled Children with WISC-R VIQ-PIQ Discrepancies of a Given Magnitude

Size of V–P Discrepancy (Regardless of Direction)	Professional and Technical	Managerial Clerical, Sales	Skilled Workers	Semi-Skilled Workers	Unskilled Workers	Total Sample
9	52	48	48	46	43	48
10	48	44	43	41	37	43
11	43	40	39	36	34	39
12	40	35	34	31	29	34
13	36	33	31	28	26	31
14	32	29	29	25	24	28
15	29	25	26	21	22	24
16	26	22	22	19	19	22
17	24	19	18	15	16	18
18	20	16	16	14	15	16
19	16	15	13	12	14	14
20	13	13	12	10	13	12
21	11	11	8	9	10	10
22	10	9	7	7	9	8
23	8	8	6	6	8	7
24	7	7	5	5	6	6
25	6	6	4	4	5	5
26	5	5	3	3	4	4
27	4	4	2	2	3	3
28–30	3	3	1	1	2	2
31–33	2	2	<1	<1	1	1
34+	1	1	<1	<1	<1	<1

From Kaufman, A. (1979). *Intelligent testing with the WISC-R*. Copyright © by John Wiley & Sons, Inc. Reprinted by permission of John Wiley & Sons, Inc.

PSYCHOLOGICAL EVALUATION

children with learning disabilities, examiners should be careful not to "overinterpret" WISC-R profiles.

K-ABC Simultaneous-Sequential Processing Differences and Subtest Scatter

There is less history of misuse of the K-ABC than of the WISC-R in the diagnosis of learning disabilities. This situation is, of course, due in part to the more recent introduction of the K-ABC. In addition, because the K-ABC contains both a measure of intellectual ability (represented by the Sequential Processing, Simultaneous Processing, and

TABLE 4-3
Percentage of Nondisabled Children Obtaining Scaled-Score Ranges of a Given Magnitude

	Regular WISC-R (10 Subtests)			Entire WISC-R (12 Subtests)		
Scaled-Score Range	Verbal (Five Subtests)	Performance (Five Subtests)	Full Scale (10 Subtests)	Verbal (Six Subtests)	Performance (Six Subtests)	Full Scale (12 Subtests)
0	100.0	100.0		100.0		
1	99.9	99.9	100.0	99.9	100.0	
2	97.5	98.6	99.9	99.0	99.6	100.0
3	86.2	92.3	99.6	94.0	97.0	99.9
4	66.7	81.1	97.0	82.1	88.5	99.3
5	45.6	64.1	89.8	62.2	74.9	95.8
6	27.3	45.6	74.7	43.2	57.0	85.9
7	14.3	29.1	56.4	25.9	39.9	70.4
8	6.4	18.0	38.6	13.7	25.9	56.8
9	2.7	10.1	22.6	6.4	14.6	32.9
10	1.2	5.2	12.3	3.0	8.1	19.6
11	0.3	2.6	5.9	1.4	4.1	10.8
12	0.2	1.4	2.9	0.4	2.1	5.3
13	0.0	0.6	1.4	0.1	0.8	2.1
14		0.4	0.5	0.1	0.4	0.6
15		0.1	0.2	0.0	0.1	0.2
16		0.0	0.0		0.0	0.0
Median	4	5	7	5	6	8
Mean	4.5	5.5	7.0	5.3	6.1	7.7
SD	1.9	2.3	2.1	2.0	2.3	2.1

Note: Scaled-score ranges equal children's highest scaled score minus their lowest scaled score on the Verbal, Performance, or Full Scales. Since scores can range from 1 to 19, the maximum possible range equals 18 points.

From Kaufman, A. (1979). *Intelligent testing with the WISC-R*. Copyright © by John Wiley & Sons, Inc. Reprinted by permission of John Wiley & Sons, Inc.

Mental Processing Composite scores) and a measure of academic achievement (represented by the Achievement subtests scores), examiners using the test are more likely to rely on the discrepancy between abilities in these two areas to make the diagnosis of learning disabilities than to make the mistake of relying solely on cognitive subtest profiles or on the discrepancy between Simultaneous and Sequential Processing scores.

Examiners using the K-ABC should, of course, be aware of the amount of difference needed between the Simultaneous and Sequential Processing scores to reach statistical significance (i.e., the level needed to be confident that differences are not due to chance). A table in the test manual provides standard score differences required for significance at each age level. The average difference required for significance for children between 2 years 6 months and 5 years of age is 14 points ($p < .05$), whereas an average difference of 12 points is required for children between 5 and 12 years 6 months. As with the WISC-R VIQ-PIQ discrepancy, a statistically significant discrepancy is not necessarily an abnormal one. The average difference between Simultaneous and Sequential Processing scores is 12.3 points. Kaufman and Kaufman (1983) suggest that a 22-point discrepancy between Simultaneous and Sequential Processing "is unusual and denotes marked scatter" (p. 194).

As described earlier, research has provided inconsistent data regarding the size and direction of VIQ-PIQ discrepancies for children with learning disabilities. Research conducted so far with the K-ABC has been more consistent in demonstrating a difference between the Sequential and Simultaneous Scales for children with learning disabilities, with Sequential Processing standard scores averaging 2 to 5 points higher than the Simultaneous Processing scores. Further analysis has shown that children with learning disabilities "performed consistently well on Gestalt Closure, one of the purest measures of Simultaneous Processing" and "tended to score most poorly on the Sequential Processing subtests" (Kaufman and Kaufman, 1983, p. 139).

Subtest scatter (i.e., the amount of discrepancy *among* individual subtest scores) was explored by Kaufman and his colleagues. The data from these studies were not available, however, at the time the manual was written.

Stanford-Binet Subtest Scatter and Discrepancy Among Areas

As is the case with the WISC-R, the Stanford-Binet does not appear to result in a "learning disabilities profile." Although the developers of the test do not discuss this issue, results from a sample of 227 children with learning disabilities is presented in the *Technical Manual* (Thorndike, Hagen, & Sattler, 1986). The largest mean difference between any of the four areas measured (Verbal Reasoning, Abstract/Visual Reasoning, Quantitative Reasoning, and Short-Term Memory) was between Verbal Reasoning and Short-Term Memory, and it was only 4.4 points. For an individual, a 4.4 point discrepancy between these two areas would not be significant. Thus, the differences among area scores does not appear to be useful in distinguishing children with learning disabilities from other children. The test developers do not discuss whether a greater amount of subtest scatter is obtained by children with learning disabilities versus other children.

Common Subtest Patterns Among Children with Learning Disabilities

As described earlier, data obtained from cognitive profiles alone are not sufficient to make the diagnosis of learning disabilities. There are, however, several patterns that often show up in test protocols of students with learning disabilities. These patterns are not, however, sufficient to make a diagnosis of learning disability, attention deficit disorder, or other developmental disabilities. They are described here simply to help professionals understand possible difficulties that may underlie or exacerbate the condition of learning disability.

In looking for patterns within the subtest profile, one must keep in mind that, because of error of measurement, a subtest score that is one or two points below another subtest score may not represent a meaningful difference in abilities on the two tasks. Kaufman (1979) suggests an easy method for determining significant strengths and weaknesses within an individual's WISC-R profile. A similar method for determining significant strengths and weaknesses within the K-ABC profile is described thoroughly in the K-ABC Manual. Examiner's using the K-ABC should rely on this method for interpreting K-ABC results. The Stanford-Binet's *Examiners Handbook* (Delaney & Hopkins, 1987) includes a chart for interpreting strengths and weaknesses within the profile (p. 87). The "inferred abilities and influences" identified within the profile are, however, based on "the judgment of the authors of this *Handbook* and their interpretation of research literature" (Delaney & Hopkins, 1987, p. 85), and the validity of these interpretations remains questionable. Delaney and Hopkins recommend that inferences based on subtest strengths and weaknesses be confirmed or denied using qualitative data regarding the child.

In reviewing the WISC-R profile, the examiner should first find the mean of the Verbal subtest scores. Next, any Verbal subtest scores that are 3 or more points above this mean should be identified (these are the relative strengths) as well as any subtest scores that are 3 or more points below the mean (these are the relative weaknesses). This procedure should be repeated for the Performance subtest scores. In using this approach, it is clear that, for example, a subtest score of 10 may indicate a strength for one child, but may indicate a weakness for another child. It is only the relative position of the subtest scores, not their absolute value, that is of interest in determining profile strengths and weaknesses.

In discussing patterns of strengths and weaknesses, Kaufman (1979) suggests that significant strengths and weaknesses be examined in combination with the other scores that are relatively high or low for the individual. For example, the first pattern to be discussed, Excessive Distractibility, is dependent on three subtest scores: Arithmetic, Digit Span, and Coding. To say that this pattern exists for a particular child, it would be necessary for the score on one of these subtests to be identified as a significant weakness, and for the score on each of the other two subtests to be below the mean for its respective group of subtests (i.e., Coding would have to be below the mean of the Performance subtests and Arithmetic or Digit Span would have to be below the mean of the Verbal subtests). Kaufman emphasizes that the patterns thus identified simply provide hypotheses for understanding the child's actual strengths and weaknesses. The examiner uses the identified patterns in conjunction with other information known about the child (e.g., from observation during testing, interviews with parents and teachers, results from other evaluations). It is recommended that the psychologist responsible for interpreting the WISC-R data familiarize him- or herself with Kaufman's (1979) approach for identifying patterns of strengths and weaknesses.

As noted earlier, several patterns appear frequently in the subtest profiles of students with learning disabilities. Again, it must be stressed that these patterns are not to be used to determine whether learning disabilities exist, but simply to help the examiner better understand the nature of any learning disabilities once they have been identified properly. The patterns described in the following paragraphs are ones the authors have seen frequently in children with learning disabilities. They are by no means unique, however, to the child with learning disabilities.

EXCESSIVE DISTRACTIBILITY. The WISC-R subtests contributing to a pattern that suggests excessive distractibility are Arithmetic, Digit Span, and Coding. The K-ABC subtests that are useful in diagnosing distractibility or short attention span are Magic Window, Face Recognition, Hand Movements, Number Recall, Word Order, and Spatial Memory. When this pattern of weaknesses is seen, the examiner should question parents and teachers about possible evidence of attention-deficit hyperactivity disorder at home and in the classroom. The examiner also should take special care to report any observation of distractibility or short attention span noted within the testing situation. It is not unusual, however, for students who appear to be attentive in the testing situation to have serious attention problems in the classroom. These children often demonstrate weaknesses on the subtest profiles for excessive distractibility, even when they do not exhibit attention problems in the one-on-one testing situation.

PLANNING ABILITY. A pattern of weakness on the WISC-R Picture Arrangement and Mazes subtests suggests that the student works somewhat impulsively, not taking time to plan before approaching a task. Especially on the Mazes subtest, a child who approaches a task impulsively will make many errors that, on this task, cannot be corrected after the student recognizes them. Although Kaufman does not list planning ability as one of the subtest patterns to be observed on the K-ABC, the examiner might observe signs of poor planning ability in the child's approach to the Photo Series subtest.

VERBAL EXPRESSION, VERBAL CONCEPT FORMATION, ABSTRACT THINKING. Many children with learning disabilities, especially those from upper socioeconomic groups, have relatively good verbal skills, as measured by the WISC-R Comprehension, Vocabulary, and Similarities subtests. Skills measured by these tests can be practiced in the context of everyday experiences (e.g., listening to adult conversations, asking and answering questions, discussing), and do not rely heavily on "school learning," especially in the younger grades. As the child with learning disabilities gets older, however, there is sometimes an observed drop in Vocabulary skills, because more of one's vocabulary is derived from reading as one gets older. (Similarly, a drop in the Information subtest score is often seen as the child with learning disabilities grows older.)

On the K-ABC, the verbal expression pattern involves the Magic Window and Gestalt Closure subtests of the Mental Processing Scale, plus the Expressive Vocabulary, Faces & Places, Riddles, and Reading/Decoding subtests of the Achievement Scale.

PERCEPTUAL ORGANIZATION. A pattern of relative strengths on those subtests that measure visual-spatial perception and organization (WISC-R Picture Completion, Picture Arrangement, Block Design, Object Assembly, and Mazes; or K-ABC Hand Movements, Gestalt Closure, Triangles, Matrix Analogies, Spatial Memory, and Photo Series) often is seen in children with learning disabilities. It should be noted, however, that this pattern also is often observed on the WISC-R for children without learning disabilities, but from impoverished environments. As discussed previously, many of the skills measured on the WISC-R Verbal subtests are those which are encouraged by discussion with adults, listening to adult conversation, asking and answering questions, and so forth. In environments where the amount and quality of language stimulation is limited, Verbal subtest scores may be artificially deflated, thus causing many of the Performance subtest scores (which are less influenced by environmental stimulation) to appear as relative strengths.

VISUAL PERCEPTION OF ABSTRACT STIMULI. A pattern of weakness on the WISC-R Block Design and Coding subtests or on the K-ABC Triangles and Matrix Analogies often is seen in children with learning disabilities, especially those whose disability appears to be due to weaknesses in spatial perception, not auditory processing. It is speculated that these are the children who often continue to reverse letters and words long after their peers have stopped, and have difficulty recognizing visual configurations of words that cannot be "sounded out" (e.g., often confusing *though*, *tough*, *through*, and *thorough*).

ABILITY TO REPRODUCE A MODEL. A pattern of weakness on the WISC-R Block Design and Coding subtests also can indicate inability to reproduce a model. This pattern of weakness can be due to poor fine-motor skills rather than to poor ability to correctly process visual perception of stimuli. The K-ABC "Reproduction of a Model" pattern includes the Hand Movements, Number Recall, Triangles, and Spatial Memory subtests. These subtests measure ability to reproduce a model in a variety of modalities—orally, motorically, by pointing, and with manipulative materials. Fine-motor skills are less important in the K-ABC pattern than in the WISC-R pattern. Attention and memory factors are, however, somewhat more heavily tapped by the K-ABC pattern, as several of the subtests require the child to reproduce a model *from memory*.

Individual students with learning disabilities will, of course, exhibit many other patterns of strength and weakness, depending on their individual abilities, backgrounds, and educational experiences. The patterns listed are presented merely to remind the examiner of some of the most common patterns observed in students with learning disabilities so that he can be "on the lookout" for them.

Supplemental Psychological Tests That May Be Useful In the Diagnosis of Learning Disabilities

As mentioned several times, measures of both intelligence and academic achievement are essential for making the diagnosis of learning disabilities. There are, however, other tests that can be added to the psychologist's battery that may help in understanding learning disabilities after they have been identified. Tests that often are used to supplement the battery include those which purport to measure skills related to visual and auditory processing. Members of the diagnostic team must be cautioned, however, that many of these tests lack sufficient reliability or are inadequately normed. For this reason it would be inappropriate to attempt to use the profiles generated from these tests to subtype the dyslexic child or to plan remedial approaches to be used with the child. Harrington (1984) claims, in fact, "If the psychologist wishes to assess sensory process deficits at all that data will probably have to be collected informally." Tests that may provide additional, useful information include the Developmental Test of Visual-Motor Integration, the Bender Visual Motor Gestalt Test, the Benton Visual Retention Test and Memory for Designs Test, the Illinois Test of Psycholinguistic Aptitude-Revised, and the Detroit Test of Learning Abilities-Revised. Of course, projective tests also may be useful in determining whether emotional disturbance is accompanying learning difficulties.

CONCLUSION

The psychologist contributes to the interdisciplinary diagnostic process by obtaining a history of the child's difficulties (from the parents' perspective), an accurate measurement of intelligence, and supplemental information that will assist in understanding the nature of any learning disabilities that might be identified. It is important that the assessment instruments used by the psychologist are reliable, valid, and meet other specific criteria outlined in this chapter. Approach to test administration is also a critical issue, as many children with learning disabilities will exhibit behaviors that typically interfere with testing. Test interpretation for children with learning disabilities should be founded on research-based principles, not on misconceived views of the "typical" child's cognitive profile.

The interdisciplinary team must, of course, rely on test data in diagnosing learning disabilities. It is important, though, that team members understand that tests are merely instruments to assist in process of diagnosis. The data should be used cautiously and only in conjunction with information about the student that has been obtained through other sources.

CHAPTER 5

Educational Evaluation

Judith Margolis
Barbara K. Keogh

Assessment has become a major enterprise in American schools, and there are many purposes for assessing pupils and many approaches or techniques that may be used. The effectiveness and the usefulness of assessment information depends, in part, on how well the purposes and the methods are matched. For example, it would be inappropriate to use a simple screening test to diagnose learning disabilities. Similarly, it would be inappropriate to assess the vocabulary of a child with a learning disability with a test of visual-motor skills.

DIFFERENCES BETWEEN PSYCHOLOGICAL AND EDUCATIONAL ASSESSMENT

Within schools there are two major assessment approaches: psychological and educational. They differ in several important ways, and both contribute to our understanding of learning disabilities. In the preceding chapter, we discussed how the psychologist provides information regarding a child's cognitive functioning, as well as information that helps rule out other conditions and explains the nature of the disabilities. In this chapter, we will look at some of the approaches and utility of educational testing and its relation to psychological testing.

A major purpose of psychological assessment in the child with learning disabilities is to determine the level of cognitive functioning, as well as to describe the psychological processes that are thought to underlie poor academic achievement. A major purpose of educational evaluation in the child with learning disabilities is to provide a differentiated and detailed picture of the child's performance in selected subject matter areas. Thus, psychological assessments are designed to describe basic, underlying processes such as memory, verbal reasoning, and attention. Educational assessments are subject matter based, are focussed on specific achievement areas such as reading, arithmetic, and spelling, and their subskills or components, for example, arithmetic computation, word recognition. Both psychological and educational assessments are essential, as establishment of a discrepancy between ability and achievement is necessary for the diagnosis of learning disabilities.

Educational and psychological assessments typically differ in administrative conditions and procedures. Psychological tests usually are administered individually out of the classroom; educational testing often is conducted in classrooms to groups of children, although individual testing is necessary when making decisions about children with learning disabilities. Psychological testing is restricted to administration and interpretation by psychologists, is often relatively short-term and limited to a few sessions, and intelligence tests usually are norm-referenced and standardized. In contrast, educational tests frequently are administered by classroom teachers, educational evaluations tend to be ongoing and cumulative over time, and educational tests often are criterion referenced and nonstandardized.

It should be emphasized that tests are only one type of assessment, and that both psychologists and teachers regularly use a whole range of techniques, including classroom observations, interviews, rating scales, and informal measures. However, the differences in educational and psychological approaches and the kind of information gained from each underscores the importance of appropriate applications and interpretations. Effective identification and intervention planning for children with learning disabilities requires information from both. In this chapter, we focus specifically on educational assessment.

EDUCATIONAL ASSESSMENT

Information gleaned from educational assessment may be used in several ways: for determination of eligibility for special education services (one element in learning disabilities discrepancy formulae); for instructional planning and monitoring; and for providing summary information about individual children, groups of children, or school districts. Sound educational assessment should yield a comprehensive picture of childrens' performance in the major subject matter or content areas, and should provide direction for program planning, including remedial efforts and/or other special instructional requirements. It also can yield information about childrens' behavior in learning situations, and about individual differences in learning styles. Numerous specific methods or techniques commonly are used in educational assessment. In this chapter, we have selected illustrative examples of widely used tests and other assessment instruments.

Standardized Norm-Referenced Tests

A number of educational tests have been developed within a psychometric tradition, and like other psychometrically based measures, many have good technical qualities. Such tests typically represent major test construction efforts, including standardization on large samples assumed to represent the average or modal achievements of children within given age or grade groups. In general, the characteristics of standardized tests include: specified and controlled procedures for administration, including time limitations; standardized procedures for scoring; and quantitative, normative scores presented in percentiles, grade equivalents, or standard scores. The normative information allows scores for individual children or groups of children to be compared; the normative information also allows comparisons across schools, school districts, and over time. For the purpose of diagnosing learning disabilities, normative data also allow comparison of childrens' cognitive ability with their actual educational achievement.

Standardized tests may be administered individually or to groups and vary in the breadth of material covered. Some provide information across different subject matter areas, others are focussed exclusively on a single subject, for example, arithmetic or spelling. The format of many of the comprehensive test batteries allows selection of subsections that may be administered separately. Most comprehensive tests yield profiles of scores, thus affording comparisons of a given child's relative achievement in different subjects. This kind of profile provides preliminary screening information useful in identification of children with learning disabilities, as by definition, these children have discrepancies between ability and achievement. Frequently they also have discrepancies across achievement areas, so that math scores may be markedly higher than reading scores, or arithmetic computation may be discrepant from arithmetic reasoning. A sampling of achievement in different subjects allows preliminary examination of the pattern of strengths and weaknesses, and thus, provides useful information.

Standardized Achievement and Diagnostic Tests

Well-known examples of standardized achievement tests that may be administered to groups of children include the California Achievement Test (CAT), the Comprehensive Tests of Basic Skills (CTBS), the Iowa Test of Basic Skills, the Metropolitan Achievement Tests, the SRA Achievement Series, and the Stanford Achievement Tests (SAT). These comprehensive batteries are from established publishers and have been developed with sound statistical procedures, including sampling and norming considerations. Generally, they are of good technical quality and provide a range of scores. They are useful in educational assessment when the purpose is to determine relative standing of children, groups of children, and/or school systems. They do not provide detailed information about how solutions are reached or what processes or steps are used in deriving the answers. It is difficult to use information from these tests for instructional purposes, nor do they provide the kind of in-depth information necessary for the diagnosis of learning disabilities.

There are a number of standardized tests that are administered individually and which yield diagnostic data in specific subject matter areas. Such tests apply primarily to the basic skill areas of reading, math, and language arts. Well-known examples of standardized diagnostic tests for reading include: the Roswell-Chall Diagnostic Reading Test of Word Analysis Skills, the Stanford Diagnostic Reading Test, the Gates-McKillop-Horowitz Reading Test, and the Gray Oral Reading Test. The Durrell Analysis of Reading Difficulty, a test with a long history, taps 16 areas that include oral reading, silent reading, listening comprehension, word recognition, word analysis, listening vocabulary, phonic spelling of words, and visual memory of words.

A number of well developed and technically adequate tests assess educational performance across subject matter domains. The comprehensive tests are widely used in the identification of children with learning disabilities. They are administered individually, have good psychometric properties, and in some cases at least, have been normed using samples from different ethnic and language groups. Detailed reviews of many currently used assessment instruments may be found in the recent monograph, *Assessment for the 1990s* (Reeve, 1989-1990). Because they so often provide the educational component in the aptitude-achievement discrepancy formulae, three illustrative tests are described here.

Kaufman Test of Educational Achievement (KTEA)

The KTEA comes in two forms, the Comprehensive Form (CF) and the Brief Form (BF). Although the two forms have the same name, they are quite different in comprehensiveness and technical adequacy, and therefore should not be used interchangeably. Although the Brief Form is acceptable for screening, the Comprehensive Form is suggested for deriving standardized scores (i.e., percentile ranks, stanines, and normal curve equivalents) and for assessing a child's strengths and weaknesses in reading, math, and spelling. The internal consistency of the subtests is adequate, although the test-retest findings as presented in the manual likely are spuriously high since they were arrived at by combining the test results of a relatively small number of subjects (172) into two broad groups; one group for Grade 1 through Grade 6 and the other for Grade 7 through Grade 12. Bands of error for different confidence intervals are presented for math, reading, spelling, and battery composite, and range from 2 (Grade 2) to 5 (Grades 8, 10, and 12) at the 68% confidence level. A relatively high correlation between the KTEA and the Kaufman Test of Cognitive Abilities (see Chapter 4) is reported by the authors, as is a somewhat lower correlation between the KTEA and the Peabody Picture Vocabulary Test-Revised (PPVT-R). The norming procedures were exceptionally good, being stratified within each grade level by sex, geographic region, socioeconomic status, and racial/ethnic group representation. Importantly, the racial/ethnic composition of the sample closely approximates that of the U.S. population at all grades.

Peabody Individual Achievement Test-Revised (PIAT-R)

The 1989 revision of the popular PIAT retains much of the format, structure, and administrative procedures of the original tests, but is changed considerably so that it is psychometrically a better test. In addition to increasing the number of items in each subtest (Knowledge, Reading, Math, and Spelling) a Written Expression subtest has been added, and scoring procedures have been revised. The inclusion of a Written Expression subtest is in line with current concern for assessment in this domain. The new scoring procedures provide a range of options for interpreting childrens' performance in terms of interindividual and intraindividual differences. All subtests, with the exception of Written Expression, are scored objectively and raw scores can be converted to developmental scores, standard scores, and percentiles. The new Written Expression subtest is scored subjectively following directions found in the manual. The norming sample is adequate in numbers at each grade and age level and in stratification in accordance with socioeconomic and ethnic/racial proportion in the population. Interestingly, although the PIAT-R is recommended for program development and evaluation for pupils who are handicapped, no effort was made to include children in special education classes in the norming sample. Test-retest reliability reported in the manual is high for subtests and for composite scores at all ages with the exception of age 12. Internal consistency coefficients also are high. An important new addition is the inclusion of standard error of measurement (SEM) tables for all subtest and composite scores, resulting in a more precise estimate of a child's performance than was possible with the old form of the PIAT.

Validity of the PIAT-R is less well documented. In a review of the PIAT-R, Lazarus, McKenna and Lynch (1989-1990) report that those being assessed are sometimes required to respond to questions posed in a manner quite different from that commonly used in classrooms, therefore pupils may know the content but be unsure of what they are asked to do. Lazarus, et al. also criticize the reading comprehension subtest on the ground that it is not constructed to take into account contemporary conceptualizations of the reading process. Although the PIAT-R is a well-standardized test and includes a broad range of academic tasks, the test author emphasizes that the PIAT-R was not designed as a diagnostic test or as a method to provide a precise measure of the content areas addressed. Rather, the PIAT-R may be viewed better as a screening test for identifying childrens' strengths and weaknesses relevant to educational and career goals.

Woodcock Johnson Psycho-Educational Battery-Revised (WJ-R)

This revision represents a substantial modification of the original test. The cognitive battery has been revised and is reviewed in Chapter 4. Although the WJ-R usually is administered as a total battery, for the purpose of this review only the achievement battery will be discussed. The authors of the WJ-R have added 4 new tests, making a total of 14 tests, 9 of which make up the standard battery. Alternate forms are available. The norming sample was based on the most recent U.S. census data according to region, community size, sex, race, and socioeconomic status. However, stratification is not reported by age or grade level and only the timed subtests were examined for stability (test-retest reliability). For the standard battery, 46% of the age by subtests correlations reported are below the accepted level ($r = .90$). Sufficiently high reliabilities are reported, however, for the Broad Achievement Clusters, allowing the test to be used in determining an ability-achievement discrepancy. The less than adequate reliabilities for subtest scores suggest caution in using these scores for making educational decisions. The content validity of the WJ-R, based on correlations with the criterion measures (e.g., the KTEA), varies by subtest, with the bulk of coefficients in the .50s to .60s range. Similar findings are reported for the cluster scores, although the Reading Cluster correlations are, in general, more robust (r in the .80s) when compared to other reading measures. Comparison of test scores of pupils who are gifted, learning disabled, mentally retarded, and nonhandicapped yields expected differences, arguing for the validity of the test for identification purposes. It is important to note, however, that children with learning disabilities may score lower than expected on the cognitive battery of the WJ-R. This situation, of course, would affect the size of the discrepancy between aptitude and achievement as measured with the WJ-R.

Limitations of Standardized Assessment

Before discussing other approaches to educational assessment, it should be emphasized that a number of factors may affect an individual's performance. Standardized administrations, especially group tests, may present particular problems for children with learning disabilities, thus raising questions about the accuracy and the interpretability of results. For example, poor motivation, lack of interest or confidence, difficulties in understanding and following directions, and/or limited familiarity with test taking may lower performance and lead to underestimation of knowledge and skills. Time limitations also may depress the performance of children with learning disabilities. Similarly, because curricula for children with learning disabilities may differ from the instructional content provided regular education pupils, the material covered in standardized tests may not overlap the content of instruction. Although test developers attempt to separate language and reading ability from measures of arithmetic, these are not entirely independent. Thus, problems in reading may influence how a child performs on a standardized arithmetic test. These influences may be important particularly when assessing children with learning disabilities from non-majority cultural or linguistic backgrounds. The language demands may be troublesome and the content of tests may be unfamiliar, but also cultural differences in how children interact with adults, or even prior experience in test taking, may depress or distort performance.

Measurement Problems in Establishing a Discrepancy

The use of standardized tests in the identification of learning disabilities is of particular interest. Recall that a major definitional requirement in learning disabilities is a discrepancy between ability and achievement. This is a defensible distinction in theory, but one which has many practical and operational problems. Problems are due, in part, to the technical limitations of the actual tests used, including errors of measurement inherent in standardized measures, and in part to the strong association between ability and achievement. Thus, it is sometimes difficult to determine if a particular test is really a measure of aptitude and ability or of learning and achievement.

Three important factors must be considered when choosing a standardized achievement test to establish a discrepancy between cognitive ability and academic performance. These are: the reliability of the test, its validity and objectivity, and the cognitive test to which it is being compared (see Chapter 4 for discussion of cognitive tests appropriately used for identification of children with learning disabilities).

Most commonly used achievement tests have reasonably high test-retest and internal consistency scores. An important consideration, however, is measurement error. The estimated error (the standard error of measurement) is an important statistic for the test user to include in determining a discrepancy between measures. A child's actual score on any test is made up of the true score plus error. Because the true score is never known, the standard error of measurement (SEM) provides a range of scores within which the true score probably falls. Thus, if a pupil obtains a score of 72 and the SEM is 10, with a 68% confidence criterion, the true score likely falls between 62 and 82. The smaller the SEM for a particular test, the more confidence the examiner can have in the actual or obtained score. The good news in computing a discrepancy is that the SEM for most standardized achievement tests is reported in the technical manuals. The bad news is that different SEMs may apply for different ages/grades, and for different subtest or cluster scores. A given test may have a small band of error for Grade 4 through Grade 6, but have a large error band in Grade 1 through Grade 3, making it a good test for use in the upper grades but a poor choice for use with primary level children. Similarly, a particular test may have a small SEM in reading and a large SEM in arithmetic, making it a reliable test for assessing one subject but not for the other. These differences underscore the importance of careful examination of the technical aspects of a test when making decisions about individual pupils.

It is important to note, too, that discrepancy scores usually are less reliable than the scores from each of the two tests being compared. Said differently, the standard error of measurement of the discrepancy score will be larger than the SEM for either the cognitive or the achievement score. Why? Because the reliability of the difference between the scores on two tests is a function of: the reliability of test A, the reliability of test B, the correlation between tests A and B, and differences in the norming groups for each test. Let us assume that we have chosen carefully the cognitive and the achievement tests so that each has good reliability ($r = .90$). Using one of several accepted formulae for calculating the standard error of measurement of a difference score (Stake & Wardrop, 1971; Thorndike, 1963), we will find that the discrepancy score has a larger SEM than either of the two tests. We may infer, then, that the discrepancy score is more variable, has a broader band of scores, than either of the tests separately. The reliability of the discrepancy score may be improved by using more reliable tests of intelligence and of achievement, and/or by using tests normed on the same population.

A second important aspect of test selection has to do with validity. Does the test measure what it purports to measure? Does the content adequately represent the subject matter area being assessed? Are the norms appropriate for the cultural and language background of the children being tested? Selection of an educational test requires going beyond the name of the test to consider the scope and relevance of the content. Many tests have "face validity." They have the right names and the content appears appropriate, yet close examination may reveal that the items are limited in scope or may not accurately represent the subject matter presumably being assessed. A test of reading comprehension may in fact be made up of items tapping only word recognition, or a test of arithmetic reasoning may be heavily weighted with computation problems. Closely related, the validity of a test of achievment in one subject matter area may be confounded because of problems in another. For example, the accuracy or validity of an arithmetic test may be threatened because the items are presented as word problems; thus, the measurement of a child's competence in arithmetic computation may be inaccurate because of his level of skill in reading.

A test is merely a sample of behavior, and to be a valid sample it must contain a sufficient number of items to allow a judgment about a pupil's level of performance. Abbreviated tests and short forms may save administration time but result in less than adequate assessment of achievement. An example is the Wide Range Achievement Test-Revised (WRAT-R) which has only a limited number of items in each subject matter domain (reading, arithmetic, spelling). In addition, the reading section is made up of word recognition items and the arithmetic section assesses only computation. The limited content restricts interpretation, and has led to a number of challenges to the use of the WRAT-R as the achievement component in the computation of a discrepancy. Similarly, in a recent review Doll (1990) concluded that there are not enough items in the Kaufman Achievement Test at the first grade level to reliably differentiate children with learning disabilities from other delayed learners. This, of course, suggests caution in interpreting KTEA results in the early school years.

Finally, the use of tests that are inconsistent with a child's cultural and language background poses a threat to validity, as the norms for most achievement tests assume similarity of opportunity. From an applied perspective, the normative sample used in test development is an important consideration in test selection. The important point is that test results are only as good as the tests from which they are derived. Educational tests are essential in the identification and diagnosis of children with learning disabilities, and there are a number of tests that meet the requirement of technical adequacy and that provide a comprehensive picture of childrens' patterns of achievement. Tests that yield inconsistent and variable scores, that do not tap appropriate and relevant subject matter domains, or that are based on incomplete or inadequate norming samples, do not provide a solid basis for identifying children with learning disabilities. Decisions about test selection should not be made on the basis of availability and popularity, but rather should be based on the soundness of the measure, on the purposes for testing, and on the appropriateness of the test for the individuals being tested. These decisions can be made only when the tester has a thorough understanding of the test, its psychometric properties, and its limitations.

Criterion-Referenced Tests (CRT)

To this point we have focused on the use of tests to determine eligibility for learning disabilities services. Another major purpose of educational assessment is to provide information for instructional planning. Norm-referenced tests have limited utility for this purpose, and there have been a number of efforts to develop formal tests that provide closer links to school curricula. Criterion-referenced tests (CRTs) and procedures are aimed at assessing information that is closely tied to the content of instruction. Formal and commercially prepared CRTs assess skill areas generally taught in "typical" school curricula. Terminal skills are task analyzed to produce a hierarchy of subskills and arranged in sequential order so that a child can be assessed in relation to mastery of that skill. CRTs may be useful particularly in the assessment of children with learning disabilities who often have uneven profiles of learning and achievement. CRTs provide teachers with information on where in the skill sequence to begin instruction and what components to emphasize. Like other assessment approaches, CRTs differ markedly in technical adequacy, scope, and in requirement of administration.

The Brigance Diagnostic Inventories is a well known and widely used commercial CRT. There are three Brigance batteries: The Diagnostic Inventory of Early Development, for children with developmental ages under 7 years; The Diagnostic Inventory of Basic Skills, for children functioning from first through sixth grades; and The Diagnostic Inventory of Essential Skills, for use with secondary school students. Reviewers of the Brigance scales note that they are useful for assessing young children's mastery of specific educational objectives, but also note the lack of information regarding reliability and validity. The strength of the Brigance scales lies in their close links to the content of intervention and in their clinical applicability, rather than to quantitative findings they yield. Recently some of the more widely used commercially prepared CRTs have included norms so that they could be used as full-service tests to identify children with learning disabilities. These include The Multilevel Academic Survey Test (MAST) and The Basic Achievement Skills Individual Screener (BASIS).

Critique of Criterion-Referenced Tests (CRTs)

Although formal CRTs are useful in providing information on mastery of skills within broad content areas, they do have limitations. First, there are a number of different curricula in the schools, and skills are not always taught in the same sequence as presented on the test; thus it can be expected that some children will do poorly on the tests although achieving adequately in class. Second, the number of items selected is limited due to constraints of administration time; it is conceivable and likely that a child with learning disabilities might know the material in one example but not in another. When CRTs are used to examine achievement, the question of curriculum match, along with the reliability of the limited sample of items to assess skill areas, must be considered.

Curriculum-Based Assessment and Measurement

Curriculum-based assessment (CBA) is an example of criterion-referenced approach which is specific to a given curriculum or classroom instructional program. CBA procedures assess childrens' performance within the context of the actual curriculum being taught. The purpose of CBA is to identify specific instructional needs. Accordingly, CBAs may include a range of classroom-based assessment techniques, including weekly spelling or chapter review tests. While some applications of CBA are relatively unstructured and informal, the trend is toward more precise, prescribed procedures. Blankenship and Lilly (1981), Howell and Moorehead (1987), and Salvia and Hughes (1990), as examples, have developed somewhat different approaches which are based on common principles underlying CBA. First, the procedures are administered in the classroom and test items are drawn directly from the curriculum, and, therefore, are context specific. Second, the assessment is ongoing. Direct and frequent measures of a child's performance on a series of sequentially arranged objectives are charted; this information is the basis for instructional planning. Finally, the assessments are peer referenced so that data are interpreted in relation to the performance of classmates of similar age, socio-cultural, and school experience.

A well known structured approach to CBA is the Curriculum Based Measurement (CBM) system developed by Deno (Deno & Fuchs, 1987). CBM is not a test in the traditional sense, but rather it is a set of evaluation procedures which allow monitoring progress toward a specified curricular goal. The prescribed procedures specify test duration, frequency of administration, procedures for scoring, and rules for summarizing and evaluating assessment information. Both the content and the pace of instruction are modified continuously in response to the identified relationships between daily performance and anticipated progress. The validity, reliability, and objectivity of measurement is stressed in this system as in many other CBA approaches.

Strengths and Limitations of CBA

Whether formal or informal, CBA approaches differ from standardized norm-referenced tests in several important ways that are relevant to learning disabilities. The procedures are administered in the classroom and are based on the curriculum in that classroom. Assessment is ongoing and continuous (rather than semester- or year-end assessment) and information is gathered on a day by day basis. The detailed, context-based assessment data allow examination of specific skills and processes used in problem solving. Finally, the assessment data can be interpreted in relation to the performance of classmates, allowing inferences that a given child's underachievement constitutes a deficit in learning, although the reason for this deficit may not be a specific learning disability. Detailed description of CBA may be found in the November, 1985 issue of *Exceptional Children*.

Adherents of CBA argue that the approach is effective with children with learning disabilities as it pinpoints specific problem areas and allows teachers to implement different instructional approaches while systematically monitoring effectiveness. CBA proponents also suggest that many learning problems are curriculum based rather than child based, and are due to ineffective and imprecise instructional goals and methods rather than to deficits in children's abilities. These are appealing points when applied to children with learning disabilities. CBA is not without critics, however, and serious questions about its utility and appropriateness have been raised (Heshusius, 1991). Major criticisms have to do with the limited scope of CBA curricula and, thus, with the content of assessment; with the almost total control of the content and sequence of material to be learned; with the quantitative, measurement-driven emphasis; and with the lack of attention to broader and more complex aspects of learning and learning processes.

Dynamic Assessment

A growing number of psychologists and educators agree that meaningful educational assessment must focus on children's potential for change, must tap children's ability to profit from instruction. This, of course, is a very different view of assessment from the approaches already described. Although the specifics of content and techniques differ, there are several major assessment approaches that are aimed at describing children's potential for learning. These include Feuerstein's (1979) Learning Potential Assessment Device (LPAD), Brown and Campione's (1986) assisted learning and transfer program, Budoff's (1987) learning potential assessment system, and Carlson and Weidl's (1979) testing the limits approach. These approaches often are referred to under the rubric of dynamic assessment or assisted assessment, and they have in common a focus on identifying the processes used in learning rather than on the products of learning.

The purpose in dynamic assessment is to discover and describe the approach a child uses in problem solving and to aid the learner in using more effective strategies. According to Lidz (1987), dynamic assessment provides a picture of the learner's potential for cognitive development, identifies processes used in problem-solving, and yields information that can be used in instruction. The goal is not just to describe what or how much has been learned, but how, and with what kind of help, learning occurs.

Dynamic assessment may take different forms and target different skills. Some dynamic assessment procedures prescribe protocols for the examiner's role, and specify the nature and amount of help to be given during the teaching phase of the assessment. Other approaches are less structured and allow the examiner administrative flexibility. In all systems the examiner interacts with the child in a teaching-learning interchange, asking questions, and providing prompts and manipulations that lead the learner through problem-solving procedures toward a successful solution.

Examples of more structured approaches include those of Budoff (1987), Carlson and Weidl (1979), and Brown and Campione (1986).

These systems are based on some form of a test-teach-test model, beginning with an initial evaluation of a child's competence, followed by a mini teaching session, and then retesting with a series of progressively more difficult tasks. The content of assessment may be domain or subject matter specific, or may be more general and nonspecific. In each case, however, the goal is to find out whether and to what extent the pupil was able to profit from the instruction and to determine what instructional adaptations and cues were effective.

In contrast to the test-teach-test approach, Feuerstein (1979) argues for a more global approach in which the focus is on broad cognitive processes thought to underlie learning, and in which the assessment is clinical and unstandardized, individualized, and interactive. He has developed training materials that are different from school-like tasks, but it is assumed that there will be transfer if there is change in the underlying processes. In Feuerstein's approach, assessment and instruction are inseparable. The clinical nature of the LPAD makes it an attractive alternative to traditional, psychometrically based approaches. However, the lack of structure and the melding of assessment and instruction make it difficult to evaluate, and the direct impact or transfer of the training to school subjects also is uncertain.

Taken as a group, the assisted assessment or dynamic assessment models are promising ways to gather instructionally relevant information about learners. They have considerable clinical-educational utility and deserve consideration when assessing children with learning disabilities, as many such children have unique or specific processing problems. Further, by definition these children have a discrepancy between presumed aptitude and actual achievement. This discrepancy may be documented by psychometric techniques, but the functional or instructional implications are obscure. The dynamic assessment approaches, on the other hand, integrate assessment and instruction. Importantly, they allow children the opportunity to demonstrate their responsiveness to instruction, and provide some cues or hints as to the potential for further learning. The reader is referred to a comprehensive review by Campione (1989) for a detailed discussion of these approaches.

INFORMAL ASSESSMENT

Informal assessment probably is as old as teaching itself, and is accepted as an essential step in educational evaluation. Teachers use informal procedures to gather information useful in planning or modifying instruction on a day by day basis. Informal assessment procedures range from casual and unstructured to systematic and structured. Examples include weekly spelling or math quizzes, rating scales, skills inventories, checklists, or observations. Most allow for flexibility of administration and interpretation.

The case for the use of informal procedures of assessment in children with learning disabilities is particularly strong, because these children are characterized by idiosyncratic patterns of performance. Not only are they different from their normally achieving peers, they are different from each other. Their unique patterns of learning often result in gaps in knowledge and in uneven problem-solving skills and strategies. These "peaks and valleys" often are lost in the summary information provided by formal testing. Sensitive and powerful remedial planning requires detailed pinpointing of the nature of the difficulties. This kind of assessment often is carried out informally by skilled teachers, but may be systemized with the use of commercially prepared inventories, checklists, and behavior rating scales, and through observation.

Observation

Observation is a direct method of assessment because it involves documenting behavior in the context in which it occurs. This reduces the inferential leaps required in interpreting test scores, and allows a close relationship between assessment and intervention decisions. Observation techniques frequently are used to assess social and classroom behaviors of children who are learning disabled, and to identify behaviors that may disrupt or interfere with learning. Observation also may be useful in describing learning styles and problem-solving skills, and in diagnosing specific problem areas. Observations may be categorized as systematic or nonsystematic.

Casual or nonsystematic observation occurs naturally in classrooms and yields anecdotal, subjective information that can provide teachers with important diagnostic information. An experienced teacher can pinpoint problems in word analysis by observing and recording during oral reading sessions, or can identify a carrying or borrowing problem in arithmetic by watching the child attempt a series of simple numerical problems. One advantage of informal observation is that it allows the teacher to reach a tentative conclusion quickly and to try out remedial techniques, thus, reducing the chances that the errors will be repeated or the problems compounded. On the negative side, unsystematic observation may not provide a clear or complete picture of a child's problems, because the observer may be overly sensitive to certain behaviors and ignore or be unaware of others. The possible effect of bias is real when observations are unsyvstematic.

Observer bias is lessened when more systematic approaches are taken. An important aspect of systematic observation is that the procedures are preplanned, performed in an explicit, prescribed manner, and the data are analyzed objectively. There are a number of behavioral observation systems and recording forms that are available and are used appropriately with children with learning disabilities. They range from relatively brief and global "snapshots" to continuous, detailed, and comprehensive recording of specific behaviors. An example is the Critical Incidence Log (Sugai, 1985).

One of the most common methods included in systematic observation systems is frequency recording—how many times a particular behavior occurs within a specified time frame. The number and breadth of the time frame and the specific behaviors to record vary according to the nature of the problems under study. Guerin and Maier (1983) have detailed three types of observational techniques in addition to frequency recording: chronologs, sequence samples, and trait samples. All may be used by teachers in classrooms. *Chronologs* involve objective observations recorded at different times of day and in a variety of settings. Data include details about time, activity, location, and who is present. The approach is useful when attempting to determine the situations or events that elicit maladaptive behavior. *Sequence sampling* is situation based, and requires recording the conditions and behaviors that precede and follow problem behaviors. In *trait sampling* the observer identifies a global characteristic, or "trait," breaks down the characteristic into more specific and objective behaviors, and identifies specific exemplars of each category. A broad descriptor like aggression might be defined as physical or verbal, and/or as acts against persons or property. These categories in turn would be divided into specific behaviors that could be observed objectively, for example, hitting or kicking another child, swearing at the teacher, tearing up work books.

Whatever the specific method or approach adopted, we underscore the utility of observational information in understanding and planning interventions for children with learning disabilities. Systematic observations can provide an objective and differentiated picture of strengths and weaknesses. Observations conducted in the classroom provide information which link the problems to the context in which the problems occur. This is especially important for children with learning disabilities, because the inconsistencies in their skills and achievements make them particularly vulnerable to the impact of instructional techniques and to classroom organization and demands.

Inventories, Rating Scales, and Checklists

In addition to detailed behavioral observations in children with learning disabilities, impressions of children's abilities and problems often are gathered using checklists, rating scales, and inventories. Often the techniques may be used in conjunction with one another. For example, a checklist of types of errors common in oral reading might be used with an informal reading inventory, or a checklist might be used to identify problems to be targeted in classroom observation. Inventories and checklists often are subject specific. Well constructed reading inventories frequently include items that specify skills in word definition, recall of facts, main ideas, and so forth. A longtime favorite with teachers, the Informal Reading Inventory (IRI), provides guidance in determining which word attack skills have not been mastered, and it indicates whether a given pupil is at the independent, instructional, or frustration level in reading.

Subject-matter inventories may be teacher developed or commercially prepared, for example, The Analytic Reading Inventory, the Classroom Reading Inventory, or the Ekwall Reading Inventory. They all provide a direct and relatively simple way of describing childrens' component skills or problem areas. One limitation is, of course, that the components identified are restricted to those contained in the particular inventory, thus important aspects of a learning problem may be overlooked. In addition, the accuracy of the information may be affected by the level of the teacher's experience and knowledge of the subject matter.

Rating scales commonly are used to describe behavioral indicators of problems such as inattention, inability to follow directions, poor social skills, and other personal, even stylistic characteristics. Rating scales are sometimes used as a way of monitoring the effects of medical interventions (e.g., stimulant medications with children with attention-deficit hyperactivity disorder) or of behavior-modification programs. Like inventories and checklists, rating scales can be useful in educational evaluation, but they also are restricted by the range or scope of content covered and by potential inaccuracies related to rater bias or to limited knowledge of the pupil and/or situation. Examples of widely used and psychometrically well founded scales are the Quay-Peterson Behavior Problem Checklist, the Achenbach Child Behavior Checklist, and the Barkley and Edelbrock School Situation Questionnaire.

CONCLUSION

Educational assessment is an integral component in the aptitude-achievement model commonly used for identifying children with learning disabilities. Standardized, norm-referenced tests are used appropriately for this purpose provided they have adequate psychometric and technical properties, and that they are individually administered. Educational assessment has another major purpose, that is, to provide information that leads to appropriate and effective intervention. In our view there are two aspects of "testing for intervention." One is the demonstration of a child's maximum performance, so that we learn what the child can do, not just document what he or she cannot or does not do. The second is to identify the context or conditions in which successful learning occurs. The first goal implies assessment with appropriate and technically adequate instruments and techniques, assurance that the methods and procedures of administration and data collection are adequate, and that the conditions of assessment are positive. The second implies the need to consider a broad range of possible influences on childrens' performance, including assessment of the physical, social, and educational characteristics of the classroom and of the instructional program. Different approaches to assessment are available, and there is a plethora of specific techniques. The challenge in assessment is to be sure that the purposes and the methods match.

CHAPTER 6

Language Evaluation

Doris J. Johnson

In Chapter 1, we introduced the idea of primary (neurologically based) handicapping conditions, which include learning disabilities and attention-deficit hyperactivity disorder. In this chapter, focus is on primary handicapping conditions in speech-language. A comprehensive study of oral language is an essential part of any evaluation of children with learning disabilities, from preschool through adulthood. Since auditory language is the first symbol system that a child acquires, any serious delays usually are noted early in life by family, physicians, and others. Mild to moderate problems, however, may not be detected until the child enters school and is expected to understand verbal instructions and convey ideas in more specific ways. Language competence is critical in school because most instruction in new subject matter such as reading, writing and mathematics is delivered orally. Furthermore, reading and writing development depend upon good underlying vocabulary, syntax, and linguistic awareness. Thus, any academic problem may be a reflection of more basic problems in oral language.

The language evaluation should occur in conjunction with other components of the psychoeducational and neurodevelopmental assessments, because there are many reasons for language problems. Delays of language development can occur as a result of peripheral hearing impairments, as a manifestation of diffuse cognitive dysfunction (i.e., mental retardation), as an expression of emotional disturbance and/or psychosocial deprivation, or as a specific deficit of expressive and/or receptive language development (i.e., a true communication disorder).

To rule out delays of language development resulting from peripheral hearing impairments, every individual with suspected problems should have a complete audiological evaluation. To rule out language delays arising within the context of mental retardation, assessment must include appropriate tests of mental ability (both verbal and nonverbal). Psychosocial deprivation and/or emotional disturbance should be assessed through the family and school history, specifically focussing on adequacy of linguistic exposure and other factors that might relate to the child's emotional development.

The person with a true communication disorder will have adequate hearing, at least average nonverbal cognitive ability, and history of adequate linguistic exposure and psychosocial environment. Although these individuals appear to have relatively specific deficits in language, they rarely have only verbal deficits. Associated deficits may include difficulties with gesturing, drawing (Cicci, 1978), symbolic play (Cable, 1981), hypothesis testing (Kamhi, Catts, Koenig, & Lewis, 1984), classification tasks (Friedman, 1984), and with other forms of representation and symbolic processes. Therefore, the evaluation should include a study of all areas of symbolic behavior including reading, writing, mathematics, music, and foreign languages to determine the breadth of the problem. Nevertheless, the focus of this chapter is on oral language, both expressive and receptive.

APPROACHES TO ASSESSMENT

There are various ways of studying language; however, several general issues should be considered. First, all language is rule governed. Therefore, the evaluation should include an investigation of each rule system to determine whether there are problems at the level of rule acquisition, application, or automaticity. Second, because children with learning disabilities have problems processing information normally, the language evaluation should include several measures of receptive and expressive language components to determine why the person is not acquiring the rules. This situation means that one cannot rely on verbal output as an indication of what children know. For example, children with serious expressive disorders may have excellent comprehension, but cannot retrieve or access words they want to say. Others have the ability to repeat words and sentences but cannot understand. Therefore, we study both receptive and expressive aspects of each rule system. These aspects will be discussed later in the chapter.

Another general issue to consider is that all tests assess multiple functions (Johnson, 1983). Even though a test purports to measure a specific function such as discrimination, memory, or retrieval, usually several subskills are required. Hence, a failure can result from several factors. For example, errors on a picture vocabulary test may be due to verbal deficits as well as problems with picture interpretation.

Finally, language assessment should include both standardized tests as well as observations in naturalistic settings. Although test scores may be requisite to document eligibility for services, many meaningful aspects of language may be assessed more appropriately in less formal settings, for example, through observation of language interactions with parents, peers, and others. For example, the child with psychosocial deprivation may appear to be relatively noncommunicative in the formal test situation, but may communicate in an age-appropriate fashion when relating to peers in a play situation. Information gained through such informal observation may be very important in the diagnostic and remediation processes. The remainder of this chapter is devoted to discussion of both formal and informal methods of language assessment.

RULE SYSTEMS

There are several rule systems that children must acquire to use language. One is phonology or the rules that govern the organization of sounds in the language. Problems in phonology typically result in faulty articulation, which may be of receptive origin (poor auditory discrimination) or related to expressive production. Although all children with learning disabilities do not demonstrate articulation problems, children with articulation problems should be watched carefully for potential problems in reading and spelling. The assessment should, therefore, include formal tests of articulation, as well as informal assessment of spontaneous speech.

A second rule system is syntax or the grammar of the language. This refers to the organization of words in sentences. Children with severe syntax problems may use single words but not understand the relationships between words. Consequently they may speak in telegraphic language (e.g., Mom - me - go - store). Those with milder problems may have difficulty with subject-verb agreement or formulation of complex sentences. The evaluation typically includes tasks such as sentence repetition (with increasingly complex sentences), spontaneous language examples to elicit various sentence and question forms, sentence building (using a specific word in a sentence), sentence combining, and various naturalistic tasks. From these samples, the clinician uses developmental norms to determine whether the child is progressing normally and/or whether there are specific error patterns.

Morphology, often considered a part of syntax, is the rule system used for plurals, verb tense and forming derivations (e.g., apply, application). Many children with language-based learning disabilities have difficulty with this rule system, particularly in written language. During testing they are asked to respond to statements such as "show me the boy, or the boys" or they are asked to complete sentences (e.g., "This boy is jumping; yesterday he _____.") Older students may be given nonsense words such as "troppy, troppier, _____" to evaluate their rule application.

Semantics is concerned with the meaning of language, or "what means what." In English, children must learn that the same word may represent a wide variety of objects and experiences. For example, "bill" can represent a person, a part of a bird, a piece of paper, or an action. Learning language is not simply a matter of forming simple associations. Rather, according to Bowerman (1976), words are "tags for concepts." Thus, when assessing semantics we must be concerned about the individual's conceptual skills, the ability to abstract critical attributes and draw inferences. Often individuals are asked to sort or classify objects and tell how they are the same. Individuals with language disorders may be able to sort but not give a good explanation. Others have problems with both classification and language.

With increasing age, children are expected to understand more complex vocabulary and figures of speech. In addition, they must comprehend more lengthy units of discourse such as lectures and stories. Expressively, they must retrieve and organize words to convey meaning to others. The assessment includes a study of comprehension of single words, sentence and discourse comprehension, as well as expression.

Finally, we investigate pragmatics or the rules of language usage. This usage includes conversational skills, turn taking, and the selection of language that is appropriate for the situation. Various aspects of nonverbal communication also are included in pragmatics such as eye contact, gesture, and body language. Studies of children with learning disabilities indicate they have numerous problems in pragmatics, many of which interfere with social interaction (Bryan, Donahue, & Pearl, 1981). Because there are few formal tests for pragmatics, most clinicians observe, tape record, and videotape the individual in various real world settings and then use checklists to note specific behaviors. Some use referential communication tasks where barriers are placed between the speaker and listener to see if the individuals can convey meaning appropriately.

Halliday (1975), Wiig and Semel (1984), and others state that language is used for many purposes including giving or sharing of information, interpersonal functions, controlling, persuading, and for intrapersonal reasons such as imaging and problem solving. Therefore, we examine the ways in which the individual uses language at home, at school, and in social situations.

As stated earlier, our approach includes a study of learning processes as they interact with one or more rule systems. That is, we attempt to determine whether an individual has difficulty perceiving, comprehending, remembering, organizing, producing, or applying features of the rules. The remainder of the discussion focuses on these processes and the ways in which they might interfere with language acquisition and communication.

AUDITORY PROCESSES

Auditory Discrimination

In the area of auditory receptive language, we first note whether the person perceives sounds and words normally. We are concerned with phonemic discrimination; that is, the ability to distinguish those sounds that signal a meaning change in our language. For example, a person learning English must be able to distinguish between voiced and voiceless sounds to understand words such as "cap" and "cab" or "bit" and "bid."

Various measures are used to assess phonemic discrimination. Young children frequently are given pictures and are asked to point to the one named by the examiner (e.g., ship or chip). Older children are given pairs of words that vary by only one phoneme and are asked to tell if they sound the same. In all cases, the diagnostician must consider the cognitive requirements of such tasks and other possible reasons for failure. For example, picture discrimination tests require the integration of what one hears with what one sees. In contrast, tests that require the child to tell whether two words are the same assume an understanding of likenesses and differences. Thus, failures may result from disturbances other than discrimination per se.

Rate of perception also may be a significant factor. If words are said slowly, certain children can distinguish all of the sounds in words but they cannot process rapid speech.

The relationship between auditory discrimination and higher levels of learning are not always clear. If the problems are severe, children may have serious comprehension problems. In other cases they may misinterpret words, particularly unfamiliar ones. For example, an 8-year-old was asked, "What is the difference between a calf and a colt?" He answered, "A calf is something you put on a broken arm and a colt is something you wear outdoors." Other children may misarticulate or misspell words they fail to perceive. For example, an adult asked if we would "berify" his credentials. When asked if "verify" and "berify" sounded the same, he said "yes." Some children with discrimination problems perform quite well in reading if they have good visual perception because the visual pattern seems to stabilize the auditory. On the other hand, if they have both auditory and visual perception problems, reading also may be impaired. In clinical teaching, we utilize a child's strengths to facilitate learning through weaker channels.

Auditory Verbal Comprehension

Comprehension is the next major level for assessment. As indicated previously, some students fail to understand words because they do not perceive them correctly; others perceive and may even repeat words but do not comprehend.

To determine whether children have a disturbance of verbal comprehension, they are given tasks that require the interpretation of words, but do not demand a verbal answer. If oral responses are required, it is difficult to determine whether a failure is due to receptive or expressive problems. Moreover, children who repeat without understanding (echolalia) can be deceptive because they appear to comprehend more than they do. For this reason, statements such as the following are presented: "Show me the chair," "Put your hands under the table," "Show me the furniture," "Point to those that are made of metal." The diagnostician tries to determine which classes of words the child does or does not understand. Some tests are designed to assess various word classes, but clinicians also can prepare criterion-reference tests or informal tasks using the vocabulary from various textbooks.

Some children understand single words, but are unable to grasp the meaning of connected language. Hence, tests are selected to assess sentences of varying length and complexity. Our experience suggests that comprehension is one of the most critical portions of the evaluation but is often the least assessed. At the upper age levels, we find many children understand conversational language, but they fail to understand superordinate terms or words that refer to groups of objects or experiences (e.g., appliances, vegetables). Failures typically result in poor reading comprehension and performance in subjects such as science and social studies. Certain aspects of mathematics also may be difficult because of complex vocabulary and multiple meanings (e.g., times, borrow, set). We investigate students' ability to understand the language of instruction at school or on the job and their ability to listen and understand lectures of the type they might have in more advanced classes.

Auditory Memory

The next area for study is auditory memory span. Now we ask, "How much can the auditory system hold and for what length of time?" While it is clear that memory is required for comprehension, we see many children and young adults whose primary problems are in retention of language. Some of these students fail in school, not because they are unable to complete the work, but because they cannot remember series of oral directions. Older students have problems taking lecture notes in class. Young adults with auditory memory problems also report difficulties at work. If they do not write the directions they have been given, they frequently forget, and as a result, are reprimanded repeatedly. Some have lost jobs because they were embarrassed to write the instructions. Assessment typically involves tasks such as oral directions that do not require verbal output. We do not use digit span or sentence repetition tasks for a measure of receptive memory span because of the expressive demands.

Retrieval

In the previous section, our concern was with auditory memory at the level of recognition; however, we also investigate recall. People with retrieval problems cannot remember words they want to say even though they can understand and repeat them. In an attempt to communicate, the individual with word retrieval problems (dysnomia) may use gesture, circumlocutions, hesitations, or word associations. Young children often develop elaborate pantomime, though some also are deficient in their use of nonverbal symbols. Older students become adept at circumventing their problems by using an overabundance of nonspecific words such as "what-cha-ma-call-it" and "stuff."

In the evaluation, we look for a discrepancy between the ability to comprehend, to repeat words, and to retrieve them spontaneously. Typical tasks are: (1) "Show me your shoes; show me the pencil"; then (2) "Say these words after me—shoe, pencil"; and then (3) "What is this?" Individuals with retrieval problems typically succeed on the first two tasks, but fail on the latter. Standardized tests typically include picture naming or sentence completion. Usually, the greatest problems occur when the person tries to recall very specific words such as proper nouns and names of objects.

Students with retrieval problems also may have difficulty with oral reading. Some have difficulty recalling letter names but are quick to recognize them if the teacher says, for example, "show me *s*." Older students often have a discrepancy between their oral and silent reading; they interpret what they read, but cannot recall the specific words. They can read words that they cannot retrieve spontaneously. Occasionally they read words with similar meanings. For example, a 7-year-old read "chicken" for "bird" and "buggy" for "cart." Others are aided by the printed symbol. As with all types of learning disabilities, one must note the relationships between integrities and deficits.

Auditory Sequencing

Another common problem among children with learning disabilities is an inability to remember an auditory sequence. They remember words, but not the order of sounds (e.g., animal, enemy). A third-grade girl, trying to tell about Eskimos said, "They live in Salaka-no-Alksa-no-Skala-no-I never say sounds so they fit together right." Many adults have difficulty repeating multisyllable words such as "multiplication." The diagnostician listens for errors in spontaneous language, but also evaluates auditory sequencing by asking the person to repeat words of two or more syllables. Some tests require the student to repeat words three times, as well as short phrases. It is important to include repetition tasks, because older students are reluctant to attempt words they think they might mispronounce. If they do not try to say long words, the clinician might not detect a problem. Sequencing disorders frequently interfere with reading and spelling, particularly the latter. The students write words as they perceive and remember them. Again, however, some students improve in auditory sequencing as they learn to read. The visual image helps them remember the order of sounds. Others have generalized problems in sequencing. Some sequencing problems also interfere with syntax. Therefore, it is helpful to try to determine whether grammatical errors occur because of comprehension, memory, sequencing, or rule-application problems.

Various tasks are used for studying syntax. For example, Vogel (1974) used (1) recognition of melody pattern, (2) recognition of grammaticality, (3) comprehension of syntax, (4) sentence repetition, and (5) syntax and morphology. Most standardized tests measure one or more aspects of syntax, but it is important to obtain various spontaneous language samples as well (Wren, 1980). For example, depending upon the age of the person, one might ask the individual to recount an event, tell how to make or do something, or tell a favorite story. The diagnostician transcribes and analyzes the language to determine whether the person has made significant errors.

Oral Formulation of Ideas

The last major area of auditory expressive language is the overall formulation of ideas. Some children acquire the vocabulary and grammar of the language, but they cannot sequence ideas properly. They have no "plan" for giving a summary, an explanation, a story, or other forms of verbal expression. In our assessment, we frequently ask the person how to make or do something such as how to play a game or tell a story about a sequence of pictures. The child's language is tape-recorded so that it can be analyzed for all of the auditory processes that have been discussed here. In addition, stories may be analyzed using procedures for story grammar from Applebee (1978), Stein and Glenn (1979) and others. Many students with learning disabilities fail to include all of the relevant information. Others have the general idea but do not elaborate on it.

CONCLUSION

Language evaluation in children with learning disabilities is designed to study many levels of input and output. The clinician attempts to do a "systems analysis" to plan remediation. We investigate the student's overall communicative functions and then analyze receptive and expressive components of each rule system to determine why the person is not acquiring or using language normally. Intervention is designed to highlight the features of the rules the person is not learning implicitly. Instruction in each area is provided so the person can use rules automatically and can use language for many purposes.

CHAPTER 7

Occupational Therapy Evaluation

Winnie Dunn

Occupational therapists address activities of daily living, work, (including school work for children) and play/leisure as the necessary and desired outcomes for an individual's performance. The occupational therapist analyzes these areas by considering the contribution or barrier created by specific sensorimotor, cognitive, and psychosocial aspects of performance. Table 7-1 contains a list of common referral complaints addressed by occupational therapists.

OCCUPATIONAL THERAPY IN THE SCHOOLS

Occupational therapists work in schools to support educational outcomes. They accomplish this by identifying performance and environmental characteristics and creating opportunities that facilitate successful educational outcomes. The interdisciplinary team structure supports these activities.

When occupational therapists work in schools, they have an obligation to provide services within an educational framework. P. L. 94-142 designates occupational therapy as a related service within educational settings. This designation means that occupational therapy is provided as it is needed to facilitate educational outcomes; other valid occupational therapy concerns that do not affect educationally relevant outcomes are dealt with in other settings.

Occupational therapists employ both screening and more comprehensive assessment procedures to evaluate children who are suspected

TABLE 7-1

Common Referral Complaints Addressed by Occupational Therapists When Serving Students with Learning Disabilities

Gross Motor
Weaker than others
Unable to hop, skip, jump, run as others do
Movements are stiff and awkward
Confuses right and left
Bumps into furniture when walking around
Difficulty with dressing (e.g., donning jacket)

Postural Control
Slumps in desk
Holds head in hands
Hangs on furniture, other people for support
Fidgets in seat

Fine Motor/Visual Motor
Unable to cut
Difficulty manipulating objects (e.g., blocks)
Immature, unusual pencil grasp
Very tense pencil grasp
Weak pencil grasp, drops pencil frequently
Poor writing, coloring—light or too dark, poorly controlled
Cannot stay on the lines when writing
Cannot complete work in a timely manner
Cannot tie shoes, button shirt
Clumsy with personal hygiene items
Difficulty with mealtime utensils
Drops objects

Sensory Processing
Withdraws from touch, sounds, movements, bright light
Touches or grabs everything
Hates being hugged
Fearful about movement
Avoids heights (e.g., climbing)
Craves movement (e.g., swinging)
Lethargic

Perceptual, Cognitive, and Psychosocial Abilities
Difficulty matching, discriminating colors, shapes
Reversals in writing
Loses place on page
Poor copying ability
Cannot follow directions
Poor attention, distractible
Does not generalize skills
Low self-esteem
Difficulty with organization, time management
Emotional outbursts

of having learning disabilities. Screening procedures frequently are employed to identify developmental problems in preschoolers that may place them "at risk" for subsequent learning difficulties. Screening procedures also may be employed when a student has been identified as having difficulty with some aspect of the school experience. Team members, including occupational therapists, review records, speak to the classroom teacher, and observe during routine activities to determine whether further assessment is necessary. When problems can be resolved with simple adaptations, there is no need to conduct comprehensive assessments; they are costly and can be an arduous experience for the student.

If screening procedures suggest that more comprehensive assessment is warranted, the occupational therapist assesses performance in the areas of school work and learning, socialization, functional communication, work, play/leisure, and other life tasks. The occupational therapist assesses the child's performance in these areas, as well as the underlying factors that enable or impede the student in carrying out the tasks. These underlying factors include sensorimotor functions, such as sensory and perceptual skills, modulation of responses to sensory input, motor planning, postural control, clumsiness/incoordination, and fine motor/visual-motor integration, as well as cognitive and psychosocial skills.

In addition to assessing the skills of the individual, occupational therapists consider the variables within the environment that support or impede task performance. The environment includes the persons and objects within the environment, the time and space needs for particular tasks, and the actual demands of the required tasks. Table 7-2 outlines the major assessment strategies used by occupational therapists to test students with learning disabilities. The formal tests available emphasize the sensorimotor systems; other areas are evaluated by skilled observation, interview, records review, and informal testing.

PERFORMANCE AREAS ADDRESSED IN THE OCCUPATIONAL THERAPY EVALUATION

Because the child's school performance depends on success in several different areas, the comprehensive occupational therapy evaluation will address performance in a variety of spheres, as discussed in the following sections (Dunn & Campbell, 1991).

Problems with School Work and Learning

There are many reasons for difficulty in learning and school work; the occupational therapist attempts to identify underlying fac-

TABLE 7-2A
Formal Tests Frequently Used by Occupational Therapists When Assessing Individuals with Learning Disabilities

		Major Areas Tested						
Test Name	Age Range	Gross Motor	Praxis	Fine Motor	Visual-Motor Integration	Visual Perception	Tactile	Vestibular
Motor-Free Visual Perceptual Test (MVPT)	4 – 8 years					X		
Sensory Integration and Praxis Test (SIPT)	4 years – 8 years 11 months	X	X	X	X	X	X	X
Test of Visual Motor Skills (TVMS)	2 – 12 years			X	X			
Beery Developmental Test of Visual-Motor Integration (VMI)	2 – 15 years				X			
Bruininks-Oseretsky Test of Motor Proficiency	4½ – 14 years	X	X	X	X			
Test of Visual Perceptual Skills (Non-motor) (TVPS)	4 – 12 years					X		

TABLE 7-2B
Other Strategies Employed by the Occupational Therapist When Assessing Individuals with Learning Disabilities

Assessment Strategy	Description
Skilled observations	The therapist observes the individual while the individual is performing functional tasks; records the features of task performance that promote or interfere with outcomes
Ecological assessment	The therapist records the features of typical performance of life routines, and then analyzes the differences between this pattern and the performance of the target individual
Interview	The therapist interviews a key person to obtain detailed information about the individual's performance abilities and difficulties; can be structured or unstructured
History taking	The therapist obtains information from checklists and interviews about the individual's development and past record of performance
Record review	The therapist systematically reviews materials which have been documented about the individual to determine salient features which might guide further assessment and intervention choices

tors that support or interfere with learning. For example, the occupational therapist might evaluate a student who has the requisite knowledge and skills, but is unable to complete written assignments. The occupational therapist may identify problems in fine motor control for writing and/or perceptual deficits that make it difficult for the student to keep the place on the page while working. These underlying factors become the focus of intervention recommendations.

Problems with Socialization

Many students with learning disabilities have difficulty with some aspects of socialization. The occupational therapist analyzes the student's interactions and the settings in which they typically occur. Factors that facilitate and impede socialization are identified so that interventions can be developed. For example, a student approaches peers easily but often cannot sustain the interaction. Upon analysis of the situation, the occupational therapist determines that difficulty generally occurs in noisy environments, suggesting that the child is unable to maintain attention to the interaction with the other noises. This observation provides the basis for intervention.

Problems with Functional Communication

Sometimes students with learning disabilities have difficulty with language and communication. Functional communication refers to the actions that support communication rather than the actual content of the messages. The occupational therapist addresses functional communication issues in collaboration with speech-language pathologists and educators. For example, successful communication requires the ability to recognize and use nonverbal cues (e.g., body posture, eye contact); this ability is a relevant aspect of communication to be assessed by the occupational therapist.

Problems with Play/Leisure

Students need to be able to make choices about desired leisure activities and have the skills to engage in these activities. The occupational therapist assesses both skill development to support play and leisure and the cognitive and psychosocial development to support appropriate decision making. Assessment leads to recommendations regarding activities that may best suit the student, as well as accommodations that may be necessary to facilitate success in these activities.

Problems with Work

Adolescents with moderate to severe learning disabilities sometimes have difficulties in work that are similar to those they encounter in school. Occupational therapists address both work preparation and work performance by examining the student's strengths and deficits and the match of these strengths and deficits to work requirements. Data obtained from this type of assessment are used to adapt the work site and provide support to students once they are placed. Home management is also a relevant priority for some students; similar strategies are used to address these work tasks.

Problems with Life Tasks

It is less common for interdisciplinary teams to select personal activities of daily living as educationally relevant outcomes for students with learning disabilities. Although tasks such as personal hygiene, bathing, dressing, and eating can be difficult for students with moderate to severe learning disabilities, these tasks are carried out more frequently at home. When parents raise these issues and the behaviors are not interfering with educational outcomes, it is appropriate to refer the family to an occupational therapist in the community.

UNDERLYING FACTORS THAT INTERFERE WITH PERFORMANCE

Although the ultimate goal of the occupational therapist is to increase the student's ability to perform functional tasks, it is the knowledge of the integrity of the underlying systems that guides individualized intervention planning. Occupational therapists use their expertise to determine the contribution or barrier produced by sensorimotor, cognitive, and psychosocial components of performance to overall success at the desired task. Interventions make use of this information by structuring situations to support students in their endeavors to learn and grow. Certain performance component problems are common for students with learning disabilities, and they will be discussed in the following sections.

Problems with the Sensorimotor Systems

The sensorimotor systems provide the mechanism by which individuals learn about and act on the environment. Visual, auditory, touch, motion, and body position information enable the individual

OCCUPATIONAL THERAPY EVALUATION 117

to create maps about the body and the environment. When these maps are disrupted due to inaccurate or unreliable information from the sensory systems, behavior and performance are affected also. Table 7-2A contains a list of the formal tests that are used by occupational therapists to assess sensorimotor integrity. One of the most comprehensive tests is the *Sensory Integration and Praxis Test* (SIPT) (Ayres, 1989), which consists of 18 subtests that evaluate skills in touch, movement, and body position, visual perception, praxis, and motor performance. Tests that contribute to the evaluation of each area are discussed in the following section.

Poor Sensory and Perceptual Skills

Some students with learning disabilities have difficulty receiving and processing sensory and perceptual information. Formal tests for assessing sensory and perceptual skills are listed in Table 7-2A. Deficits in visual perceptual skills may be observed informally in tasks such as copying from the chalkboard, writing answers in the place on the worksheet, or keeping one's place on the page. Perceptual problems may be reflected in the student's inability to follow directions, remember what has been said, and screen out environmental sounds while working.

The more basic sensory systems respond to touch, body position, and motion. These systems provide information that forms the individual's body scheme, or map of the body and how it works. Some students with learning disabilities have difficulty processing this basic sensory information, disrupting their body scheme. When the body scheme is unreliable or inaccurate, the student has difficulty using body parts to create effective responses to environmental demands. The SIPT contains specific subtests to assess the integrity of these basic sensory systems. Scores reveal a pattern of performance that is combined with other data to create a complete picture of sensory processing. The occupational therapist also assesses these areas by skilled observation of performance, through interviews, and checklists from teachers and parents (Table 7-2B). The child with a poor body scheme has difficulty holding his body in the chair, or may "hang" on the back and hook his legs around the chair legs. Information from assessment of sensory and perceptual skills will be used to design interventions that include adaption of material and tasks, as well as specific remedial activities.

Poorly Modulated Responses to Sensory Input

Most individuals have the ability to accommodate to environmental changes that occur during activities. Some students with learning disabilities have a poor ability to modulate the effects of sensory input on their performance. When a student is unable to accommodate to added sensory experiences, we describe them as hyper-responsive or hypersensitive to stimuli; when students require additional stimuli to notice or respond to the world around them, we use the term hypo-responsive or hyposensitive. Any sensory channel can be affected. The occupational therapist observes behavior, talks with the student and obtains a thorough history about responsiveness to sensation to determine the pattern of this problem. Table 7-3 contains a list of common problems that students encounter when they are either hyposensitive or hyposensitive to sensory information.

Poor Motor Planning (Dyspraxia)

Students with learning disabilities also may exhibit developmental dyspraxia (Ayers, 1980; Cermak, 1985). Students who have developmental dyspraxia have difficulty conceiving, organizing, and planning motor acts. Dyspraxia seems to be related to poor sensory processing, poor body scheme, and the resulting lack of adequate and reliable information upon which to build effective movements. The SIPT contains a set of praxis tests; the occupational therapist can gain understanding of the types of motor planning problems that exist, and can verify test findings with observations and reports. As with other sensorimotor problems, the occupational therapist uses skilled observation of performance, interviews, and developmental history to complete the picture of the motor difficulties.

Poor Postural Control

When students with learning disabilities hang on their chairs, lean on objects or persons when standing, and use external forces to keep them upright against gravity, problems with postural control are suspected. Poor postural control can have a sensory, experiential or developmental base. When a student cannot hold his own body up against the forces of gravity, he or she is ill equipped to engage in learning tasks. Classroom performance presumes the individual's ability to hold the body in place; when a student cannot do this, there is little energy left for learning. Occupational therapists perform clinical tests of postural control, observe performance in school, and interview teachers and parents to determine the role of postural control in performance.

Clumsiness/Incoordination

Students with learning disabilities can display general difficulty with gross motor coordination. This difficulty is a common referral

OCCUPATIONAL THERAPY EVALUATION

TABLE 7-3
Common Observations When Sensory Systems are Poorly Modulated

Sensory System	Over-Reactive	Under-Reactive
Somatosensory (touch)	Defensive about others touching body Reacts emotionally or aggressively to touch Avoids selected textures Narrow range of clothing choices Rigid rituals in personal hygiene Extremely negative about dental work Picky eater, especially regarding textures Avoids haircuts, hairwashing	Slow to respond Does not notice others Uses poor judgment regarding personal space
Vestibular (movement)	Insecure about movement experiences Avoids or fears movement Holds head upright, even when bending over or leaning Avoids new positions, especially of head Holds onto walls or bannisters Very clumsy on changeable surfaces, such as a field	Clumsy, lethargic Slow to respond to movement demands Poor endurance, tires easily
Proprioceptive (body position)	Tense muscles Rigidity, diminished fluidity of movement	Weak grasp Poor endurance, locks joints Tires easily, collapses Hangs on objects for support
Visual	Avoids bright lights, sunlight Covers eyes in lighted room Watches everyone when they move around the room	Does not notice when people come into the room Difficulty in finding objects in drawer, on desk, on paper
Auditory	Overreacts to unexpected sounds Easily distracted in classroom Holds hands over ears	Does not respond to name being called Seems oblivious within an active environment

complaint received by occupational therapists in the schools. Clumsiness and incoordination can interfere with the student's own learning as well as disrupt the learning of classmates. Informally, the occupational therapist will observe that these students are clumsy; they drop their materials and trip on the furniture in the room, even when the furniture is in predictable locations. (Motor tests are listed in Table 7-2A.)

Poor Fine Motor/Visual-Motor Integration

It is very common for students with learning disabilities to have problems with fine motor (use of hands to manipulate objects) and visual motor (coordination of eyes and hands for manipulation) control. These skills are necessary for many school activities and tasks of daily life. When fine motor and visual motor skills are disrupted, the student has difficulty producing work efficiently; sometimes professionals misinterpret the poor work product as indicative of poor knowledge in content areas (e.g., the student is a poor speller) or of poor motivation.

Occupational therapists analyze the student's performance, task demands, the work product, and the results of formal tests to determine the exact type of visual motor integration problems that exist. (Formal tests are listed in Table 7-2A.) Intervention recommendations focus on adapting school work to decrease the demands for visual-motor output and providing specific activities to improve visual-motor skills.

Problems with Cognitive and Psychosocial Skills

In addition to the areas outlined above, the occupational therapy evaluation provides other information relevant to understanding the child's learning difficulties (e.g., difficulties in attention, motivation, behavior, organization, self image, and generalization of learning). The occupational therapist provides support to the psychologist and special educator to identify cognitive and psychosocial ability and potential. While conducting a skilled observation in the classroom, the occupational therapist might identify behaviors that interfere with attention to seatwork, interaction skills with peers or authority figures, or coping and time management. During an individual session, the occupational therapist would record the student's ability to generalize skills to a new, but similar play situation. There are several specific areas addressed frequently by occupational therapists.

Attentional, Motivational, and Behavioral Problems

The occupational therapist analyzes the contexts within which the student fails to exhibit adequate attention and motivation. When sensorimotor factors are barriers to increased attention and motivation, the occupational therapist addresses these concerns. When the problem lies in environmental areas, such as the need to establish an effective reinforcement method, the occupational therapist collaborates with other team members to identify an appropriate strategy.

The occupational therapist also considers the role of sensorimotor skills in behavioral problems such as frustration, aggression, and withdrawal. Many environmental and task adaptations are evaluated to decrease the impact of the student's problems on performance and, therefore, reduce frustration and inappropriate behaviors. Behavior management is also a viable team alternative.

Organizational Problems

The occupational therapist addresses organizational problems by evaluating the student's perceptual and sensorimotor difficulties, by observing learning environments (e.g., disorderly desk or locker), and interviewing the student regarding management strategies that work.

Poor Self-Image

The occupational therapist uses observation and interviews to clarify self-image status. The occupational therapist contributes to interdisciplinary, collaborative decisions in this area. Sometimes adaptations are successful because they enable the student to experience a positive outcome.

Problems with Generalizations of Learning

The entire team addresses problems with generalization of learning systematically, pointing out the similarities from one situation to another so the student can learn to tap already developed skills to solve current problems. The occupational therapist creates new situations which provide opportunities to practice these generalizations, and collaborates with teaching staff to identify ways to make these opportunities available throughout the day.

CONCLUSION

Individuals with learning disabilities display a complex configuration of perceptual, cognitive, and sensorimotor difficulties. The occupational therapist evaluates the performance in many settings and assesses factors that may underlie observed deficits. These factors include sensorimotor function, sensory and perceptual skills, modulation of responses to sensory input, motor planning (dyspraxia), postural control, clumsiness/incoordination, and fine motor/visual-motor integration, as well as cognitive and psychosocial skills. By understanding the individual strengths and weaknesses of the child, as well as the environmental barriers and facilitators, the occupational therapist assists in the development of appropriate adaptations and interventions.

CHAPTER 8

Interdisciplinary Diagnosis

Elizabeth H. Aylward
Frank R. Brown, III

The previous chapters have described the methods for obtaining accurate assessments of intelligence and academic achievement, as well as other information relevant to understanding the child's learning difficulties. As stated previously, the diagnosis of learning disabilities for the school-age child is based on a significant discrepancy between a child's intellectual abilities and academic achievement. There is, however, a fair amount of controversy regarding appropriate methods for determining whether significant discrepancy exists. As discussed in Chapter 2, even more difficulty is encountered when we attempt to apply a discrepancy definition to identify learning disabilities in children who have not yet reached school age. This chapter will examine methods for integrating information from the various assessments to establish a diagnosis of learning disability.

IDENTIFYING SIGNIFICANT DISCREPANCY BETWEEN ACADEMIC ACHIEVEMENT AND INTELLECTUAL ABILITIES

Neither Public Law 94-142 nor other federal guidelines provide precise diagnostic criteria for establishing a significant discrepancy between academic achievement and cognitive expectation. Although many states and local school districts have convened committees to study this issue and have outlined procedures for identifying a significant discrepancy, there is, as yet, no universally accepted method for doing this. Cone and Wilson (1981) suggest that techniques for computing a discrepancy fall into four major groups: grade level deviations, expectancy formulae, standard score comparisons, and regression analyses. These methods or models vary in statistical rigor, and yield somewhat different results.

Grade Level Deviations

Although widely used, possibly because of ease of computation, the grade level deviation approach is the most seriously flawed. In this method, a child's score on an achievement test is compared to his or her actual grade placement. If achievement is markedly below grade level, a significant discrepancy is inferred. This is not an appropriate method for identifying children with learning disabilities. Grade level equivalents lack mathematical power, are imprecise, and are inconsistent across grade levels. The approach over-identifies slow learners and children in upper grades, while at the same time underidentifying more able and younger children. It will bar from services the bright child who is at or near grade level in academic skills, but performing significantly below cognitive expectation. Similarly, children who are slow both cognitively and academically may be mislabeled as learning disabled. This method also is inappropriate because it generally delays the identification of learning disabilities until at least second grade. If a child does not qualify for special education services until he or she is two years below grade level, the child must experience at least two years in an inappropriate learning environment before receiving any special services, which results in undue frustration and wastes valuable time. Finally, the method is inappropriate because a child who is two years below grade level in the early elementary grades clearly is impaired more seriously than the child who is two years below grade level in secondary school. Many school systems fail to make this distinction when using this method to identify learning disabilities. In our view this is an inappropriate method for determining a discrepancy.

Simple Expectancy Formulae

Expectancy formulae provide a frequently used method for determining a discrepancy. They have considerable appeal as they also are relatively easy to compute and appear to be a straightforward way of combining cognitive and achievement data. In essence, a given child's expected achievement is predicted directly from his or her age or from his or her score on an ability test. If the achievement is lower than expected, a learning disability is considered. Despite its appeal, the simple prediction method has limitations. Expectancy formulae that do not take into account regression effects lead to identification of larger proportions of brighter than duller children, and sometimes lead to misinterpretations of formal fluctuations in ability-achievement. As will be discussed in more detail in this chapter, unless regression effects are considered, expectancy formulae based directly on IQ, like grade level discrepancy methods, are inappropriate for identifying children with learning disabilities.

Standard Scores

Standard scores provide still another approach to determining a discrepancy. Standard scores provide a common metric or common scale for comparing the results of different tests. Test scores for a school district or classroom are statistically transformed to yield a score which represents the relative deviation from the average or mean. The mean in standard score distributions is zero and the variance is expressed in units of 1.00. Thus, a child who is achieving above the average for the group might have a standard score of +1 or +2; a pupil whose achievement is below the average would have a standard score of –1 or –2. These scores then may be compared directly to scores on ability tests or on other achievement tests. Applied to the discrepancy question, standard scores allow a direct comparison of scores on aptitude and achievement tests, even if the two tests have different ranges of actual scores and different standard deviations. Standard scores also provide a common scale for comparing performance levels across age or grade levels. Similar levels of ability and of achievement, as is the case with average learners or with slow learners, yield similar standard scores. Differences in standard scores suggest differences between aptitude and achievement, thus indicating a possible learning disability. The method is technically sound and yields relatively precise results. However, it also requires considerable statistical work and large samples, thus it may not be feasible for many school districts or diagnostic clinics.

A related method for computing a discrepancy involves comparing scores on ability and achievement tests using deviations from the average as measured in standard deviations. Fortunately, most test developers provide information about ability and achievement tests in standard deviation units, based on the norming samples for the tests. This approach, like the statistical procedure described previously, makes it possible to compare test scores in terms of deviations from the mean or average. Rather than transforming scores into units of one, the variance from the mean is shown as standard deviations. For example, the WISC-R or the K-ABC, described in Chapter 4, have means of 100 and standard deviations of 15. (The Stanford-Binet 4th edition has a mean of 100 and a standard deviation of 16.) When used with achievement tests that have similar means and standard deviations, it is possible to define a significant discrepancy as 1, 1.5, or 2 standard deviation differences in scores (15, 22.5, and 30 points, respectively). A child with an IQ of 100 would have to obtain a score of 85 or below on the achievement test to be considered learning disabled, assuming that a cut-off of one standard deviation was being used; a child with an IQ of 115 would have to have a score of 100 or below on the achievement test to be eligible for learning disabilities services. It should be noted that the use of standard deviations for comparative purposes assumes that the norming samples from which the standard deviations were derived are appropriate for the children actually being assessed. Standard score methods certainly are superior to grade level comparisons when identifying a discrepancy between ability and achievement. Like those other methods, however, they do not account for regression effects.

The Concept of Regression Toward the Mean

Regardless of the trait being measured or the measurement instrument being used, there is always going to be some amount of error. A test with good reliability will have less "error of measurement" than a test that is less reliable. The WISC-R, which is considered to be one of the most reliable of all psychological instruments, has a standard error of measurement of 3 points. That is, a child's "true IQ" (the average IQ that would be obtained if the test could be given an infinite number of times without any retest effects) will be no more than 3 points higher or lower than the measured IQ approximately 68% of the time (the percentage of cases falling between +1 and –1 standard deviations on a normal curve). One can assume that the more deviant a score is, the larger the error of measurement it probably contains (Campbell & Stanley, 1963). Thus, the child with an extremely high score can be considered to have had unusually good "luck" (large positive error) and the extremely low scorer bad "luck" (large negative error). Because luck is capricious, one would expect students with extremely high scores on one test to score somewhat less well on a subsequent test. Similarly, the child who was unfortunate enough to receive a very low score on an initial test can be expected to score somewhat higher on a subsequent test. This phenomenon is known as *regression toward the mean*. That is, when a particular child has a score on one test that is above or below the mean, one can expect the score on a subsequent test to be nearer to, or to regress toward, the test mean. This is especially true when scores are farther from the mean or when the test is less reliable.

When one is comparing scores on two tests (e.g., an intelligence test and an academic achievement test), the problem of regression becomes even more serious than when one is comparing scores on the same test given on two occasions. The lower the correlation between the two tests, the greater the amount of regression that can be expected. Although regression toward the mean cannot be eliminated, it can be minimized by selecting tests that have good reliability. Based on the strengths and limitations of the various approaches, many diagnosticians and statisticians recommend a regression-discrepancy approach (Cone & Wilson, 1981; Reynolds, 1984). For example, when using standard scores, regression effects are taken into account when the 10 to 15% of children with the largest discrepancies at each IQ level are identified. This ensures similar decision rules or "equal opportunity" across the IQ continuum. Estimating regression effects adds complexity, but allows more accurate decisions about discrepancies, and also guards against over- or under-representation at any IQ level. This is well illustrated when predicting Educational Quotients (EQs).

Predicting Educational Quotients

School systems have begun to take the phenomenon of regression toward the mean into account by charting predicted Educational Quotients (EQs) for children with various IQ scores. By looking at Table 8-1, it becomes clear that a child whose IQ is above average can be expected to have a lower EQ than IQ. Similarly, the child whose IQ is below average can be expected to have a higher EQ than IQ. For example, a girl with an IQ of 130, which is considerably above average, can be expected to perform very well on an achievement test, but not quite as high as the 130 score. Table 8-1 indicates that she should be expected to have an achievement test standard score of approximately 118, assuming that academic achievement has progressed at a level commensurate with her IQ. If the achievement test score is significantly below 118 (not 130), one can make a diagnosis of a learning disability (assuming that other causative factors, such as emotional disturbance or lack of educational opportunity, have been ruled out).

Regardless of the method used to measure cognitive ability and academic achievement, decisions must be made as to what will be considered a "significant discrepancy." Differences in the size of the discrepancy obviously leads to different numbers of children identi-

TABLE 8-1
Predicted Educational Quotients (EQs) for Given VIQs, PIQs, and Full Scale IQs

VIQ or Full Scale IQ	Predicted EQ	PIQ	Predicted EQ
130	118	130	115
125	115	125	113
120	112	120	110
115	109	115	108
110	106	110	105
105	103	105	103
100	100	100	100
95	97	95	98
90	94	90	95
85	91	85	93
80	88	80	90
75	85	75	88
70	82	70	85

(Predicted EQs are somewhat different for PIQs than for VIQs or Full Scale IQs because the correlation between academic achievement and nonverbal intelligence is lower than that between academic achievement and verbal intelligence. See McLeod, 1979, for a more in-depth discussion of this issue.)

fied as learning disabled. McLeod (1979) suggests a cut-off of 1.5 standard deviations. Thus, if a child's score on a test of academic achievement is 22.5 points lower than the predicted EQ, a significant discrepancy has been identified, and the diagnosis of learning disability can be made. This number, 22.5, is derived by multiplying 1.5 times 15, which is the standard deviation of most intelligence tests and academic achievement tests. In the case described in the previous paragraph, the student's standard score on the test of academic achievement would have to be 95.5 (118 minus 22.5) for her to be diagnosed as learning disabled. Some school systems may choose a cut-off of one or two standard deviations in defining significant discrepancy. The cut-off level chosen will depend upon the system's philosophy regarding learning disabilities, as well as on its ability to provide services for children identified as learning disabled.

Further Considerations in Identifying Discrepancy

Choosing the Measure of Intelligence for the Cognitive-Achievement Comparison

Even after determining which tests of intelligence and academic achievement will be administered, and the degree of discrepancy needed to constitute significance, the interdisciplinary team must decide which individual scores will be compared in making the diagnosis of learning disabilities. For children whose Verbal IQ-Performance IQ (VIQ-PIQ), or Simultaneous-Sequential discrepancy is small, it is not unreasonable to compare the WISC-R Full Scale IQ or K-ABC Mental Processing Composite standard score with the standard scores from the test(s) of academic achievement. However, when there is a large VIQ-PIQ discrepancy, several different approaches to the discrepancy issue can be justified. Take, for example, a child with a WISC-R VIQ of 85, PIQ of 115, and Full Scale IQ of 99, and a WJR-ACH Reading Cluster standard score of 85. Because of the child's significant VIQ-PIQ discrepancy, it would not be appropriate to consider the child's Full Scale IQ of 99 as an accurate representation of intellectual functioning. Therefore, it would not be justifiable to use the Full Scale IQ in determining the presence of significant discrepancy between intellectual and academic abilities.

Because reading ability is more highly correlated with verbal abilities than with visual-spatial abilities, it could be argued that the child should not be expected to be reading at a level higher than the level of the child's verbal abilities. Thus, using the VIQ of 85 alone as the measure of cognitive functioning, Table 8-1 indicates that the predicted EQ would be 91. The difference between the predicted EQ of 91 and the actual reading achievement score would be 6 points. Because this does not meet the cut-off of 1.5 standard deviation discrepancy (22.5 points), no learning disability would be identified.

It could, however, be argued just as reasonably that the mechanism that is preventing verbal skills from developing at the same rate as nonverbal (visual-spatial) skills is the same mechanism that is preventing better development of reading skills. Using this reasoning, the Reading Cluster score could be justifiably compared with the PIQ of 115. Table 8-1 indicates that an EQ of 108 would be predicted for an IQ of 115. Column 2 of Table 8-1 is used in predicting the EQ from the PIQ because the correlation between PIQ and academic achievement is approximately .5, whereas the correlation between academic achievement and either the VIQ or the Full Scale IQ is .6. The discrepancy between the EQ and the actual reading achievement score in this case is 23 points, which would be significant, if a cut-off of 1.5 standard deviations (22.5 points) is used. Thus, a learning disability would be identified. We believe that this approach is more attuned to the definition of learning disabilities outlined in Public Law 94-142, which includes disorders in "the understanding of language" as learning disabilities. Similarly, it would be justifiable to compare the score of academic achievement with the VIQ alone, if it were significantly higher than the PIQ, as the Public Law 94-142 definition includes such conditions as "perceptual handicaps."

The procedure for determining predicted EQs is not necessary if one uses the K-ABC for both measures of intellectual functioning and academic achievement, as the cut-offs for significant discrepancy between tests are provided in the manual. The K-ABC routinely requires the examiner to compare the standard scores for each of the Mental Processing Scales (Sequential, Simultaneous, and Composite) with the standard score for the Achievement Scale. Thus, a significant difference between achievement and any of the scores of Mental Processing could be an indication of a learning disability.

The K-ABC does not, however, encourage routine comparison of each of the Mental Processing scores (Sequential, Simultaneous, and Composite) with individual Achievement subtest scores, but rather with the overall Achievement composite score. Thus, the routine comparison of Mental Processing scores with the overall Achievement scale may not detect the child who is seriously delayed in only one area of academic achievement. Kaufman and Kaufman (1983) caution that the Mental Processing scores can be compared with individual Achievement subtest scores, if the number of comparisons is limited by selecting wisely the most appropriate comparisons to make, based on background information about the child. Of course, the interdisciplinary team often will want to compare the child's K-ABC Mental Processing scores with scores from achievement tests other than the K-ABC. In this case, the procedure for predicting EQs outlined earlier should be followed.

If the Stanford-Binet has been used as the measure of intelligence, it seems reasonable that either the Verbal Reasoning standard area score (SAS), the Abstract/Visual Reasoning SAS, or the Composite IQ be used as the measure of cognitive ability. SAS's from the Short-Term Memory or Quantitative Reasoning Scales do not, however, reflect broad enough abilities to justify their use as the measure of cognitive ability for the diagnosis of learning disability.

Considering Individual Subtest Scores in the Cognitive-Achievement Comparison

It is important to point out that the interdisciplinary team, in making the diagnosis of learning disability, may sometimes need to consider the individual subtest scores that go into making up the overall scores of intellectual functioning (WISC-R VIQ, PIQ; K-ABC Sequential Processing standard score, Simultaneous Processing standard score; Stanford-Binet SAS's or Test Composite) and overall scores of academic functioning (e.g., WJR-ACH Reading Cluster, Mathematics Cluster, and Written Language Cluster scores). For example, on the WISC-R, several of the subtests (Similarities, Comprehension, Vocabulary) often are considered to measure more "important intelligences" than other subtests (Information, Arithmetic, Digit Span). As described in Chapter 4, the Arithmetic and Digit Span scores can often be depressed in a child who has attention-deficit hyperactivity disorder, and the Information subtest is influenced greatly by environmental stimulation (including reading). Thus, when a child's scaled scores on Similarities, Comprehension, and Vocabulary are significantly higher than his or her scaled scores on Information, Arithmetic, and Digit Span, his or her VIQ may not be an accurate reflection of the "more important" verbal skills—abstract thinking, verbal concept formation, and verbal expression—but may be depressed by verbal skills often considered less important—auditory attention, fund of general knowledge, short-term memory. The team may want to take this pattern of scores into account when making the diagnosis. If, for example, the child with the pattern just described did not have quite enough discrepancy between the VIQ and scores of academic achievement to meet the cut-off for the diagnosis of learning disabilities, the team may want to take into consideration other data to determine if the VIQ was not depressed artificially by factors generally not considered indicators of intelligence (e.g., distractibility) and adjust the criteria for diagnosis.

Similarly, the team should take into account variability within the subtest scores that comprise the measures of overall academic achievement. For example, a child may be reading on grade level, according to the overall Reading Cluster score from the WJR-ACH. However, the child might perform three years above grade level in Letter-Word Identification (word recognition) and Word Attack (application of phonics skills), but be functioning five years below grade level in Passage Comprehension. In this case the child's overall Reading Cluster score does not adequately summarize his or her reading abilities. The interdisciplinary team should again not abide by the strict criteria established for making the diagnosis of learning disability, but should consider other data that might explain the discrepancy within reading skills.

Need for Flexibility in Diagnosis

It is imperative that professionals use the formula for identifying learning disabilities as a guideline, and not as an absolute authority. For many children, it will be just as important to take into account reports from teachers and parents, observations during testing, and other data sources before arriving at a diagnosis. In some cases, it will not be possible to find a reliable and valid test to measure the child's skill in a particular area. For example, many children perform quite well on measures of written language ability, although teachers and parents insist that the child has a great deal of difficulty when required to organize his or her thoughts in writing. Because most of the tests available for obtaining a score in written language focus on the mechanics of writing (e.g., spelling, punctuation, usage, capitalization), it may not be possible to diagnose a learning disability in written language by using test scores alone. It would be necessary in such a case for the team to take into consideration teacher and parent reports, to observe the child in a situation that requires him or her to write a paragraph, and to subjectively evaluate the child's written work in terms of content, organization, neatness, and time taken to complete it, as well as correct use of spelling, punctuation, grammar, capitalization, and so forth. Only then can an accurate diagnosis be made, regardless of the presence or absence of significant discrepancy between test scores.

It is especially important that the interdisciplinary team consider factors other than the EQ-IQ discrepancy when making the diagnosis of learning disabilities in younger children. Because academic testing in the early grades (kindergarten and first grade) is based primarily on material that can be learned rotely (e.g., letter and number identification, sight words, addition facts), it may be difficult to identify the child who will have problems with more complex processes (e.g., application of phonics rules, reading for comprehension, understanding math concepts). For these young children, it is very important that the interdisciplinary team rely heavily on teacher and parent reports.

IDENTIFYING PRESCHOOL-AGE CHILDREN AT RISK FOR LEARNING DISABILITIES

In Chapter 2 we pointed up the difficulties that arise when we attempt to use discrepancy definitions, that is, discrepancies between academic achievement and cognitive expectation, to identify preschool-age children at risk for subsequent learning disabilities. At least two approaches to early identification, each based on a discrepancy model, can be envisaged to identify preschoolers with learning disabilities. The first approach, delineated by McCarthy (1989) and the National Joint Committee on Learning Disabilities (Leigh, 1986), suggests that preschoolers at risk for subsequent learning disabilities will manifest abilities and behaviors that deviate from normative expectancies. Discrepancies between anticipated and realized developmental milestones (i.e., developmental delays), especially in the areas of language and visual perceptual development, attention span, and impulse control, and behavior, are used to identify preschoolers at risk for subsequent learning disabilities. It is our contention that this neurodevelopmental approach will identify preschoolers at risk for ongoing neurodevelopmental delays and slow academic achievement commensurate with cognitive expectation. We do not anticipate that this approach would *specifically* identify that subgroup of preschoolers who will progress to have academic achievement that is discrepant from the slow achievement projected from the neurodevelopmental delay.

A second approach to early identification might be based on identifying significant discrepancies between cognitive expectation (as measured by appropriate preschool-age cognitive measures) and what might be termed "pre-academics", that is, antecedents of subsequent academic achievement. Although McCarthy (1989) and others include the assessment of "preacademic skills" in their discrepancy definitions for preschoolers, it appears that they are referring to underlying cognitive skills that form the basis for learning (e.g., verbal comprehension and concept formation, auditory and visual attention, verbal and visual memory). We are using the term "pre-academic skills" to refer to specific skills that can be considered the first actual demonstration of academic achievement in reading (e.g., letter identification, alphabet recitation, sound-symbol correspondence, rhyming, identification of words with the same initial sound), math (rote counting, number recognition, making a one-to-one correspondence, understanding concepts such as "less than," "more than," "same as," "most"), and writing (e.g., copying geometric forms and letters, writing one's own name). In this discrepancy approach, preschoolers with learning disabilities would be identified through an extrapolation of the "significant discrepancy" definition used with school-age children, with "pre-academics" substituted for academic achievement in the discrepancy definition. The difficulty with this approach is that, to date, very few instruments have been developed that measure pre-academic skills, as we define them (e.g., the Basic Concept Scale, Bracken, 1984). Furthermore, this approach requires documentation that the child has had some exposure to pre-academic skills, either through formal preschool, parental instruction, or, at the very least, regular viewing of "Sesame Street" and other preschool television programs. While this approach would probably result in a fair number of misidentifications, we feel confident that early signs of learning disabilities could be demonstrated in at least some subgroups of preschoolers (e.g., bright children who have had several years of academic preschool exposure and who are still unable to identify their own name in writing).

To our knowledge, no longitudinal studies have been conducted to investigate the predictive value of either the neurodevelopmental or "pre-academic"/cognitive discrepancy formulations in identifying preschoolers at risk for subsequent specific learning disabilities. Pending such studies, we must conclude, as indicated earlier in Chapter 2, that identification of preschoolers at risk for subsequent learning disabilities is, at best, tentative at present.

IDENTIFYING STRENGTHS AND WEAKNESSES IN THE LEARNING STYLE

Many investigators have attempted to classify children with learning disabilities (particularly reading disabilities) according to their specific difficulties. Children with reading disabilities often are thought to fall into one of two categories. Children in the first group (sometimes called *dysphonetic* dyslexics) have difficulty with auditory processing and are unable to make accurate phoneme-grapheme correspondences, are unable to break words into their phonetic components and blend the sounds together to form the correct word, and have difficulty sequencing phonemes correctly. These children make bizarre spelling errors, unrelated to the sound of the word. Children in the second group (sometimes called *dyseidetic* dyslexics) have difficulty with visual-spatial perception and may be unable to recognize individual letters, are slow to recognize simple sight words (visual gestalts), have poor visual discrimination of words closely similar in configuration, and have trouble recognizing nonphonetically spelled words. These children read very slowly, as they must decode each word as they go along. They spell words the way they sound, ignoring irregular patterns usually learned through a sight approach (e.g., "tough" may be spelled "tuff").

Some investigators have divided children with reading disabilities into these or similar groupings based on the direction of the VIQ-PIQ or Sequential-Simultaneous discrepancy, subtest profiles from the intelligence tests, or by an analysis of reading and spelling errors. In some schools, attempts have been made to tailor the curriculum to address the strengths and weaknesses presumed to be exhibited by the different groups. Sadly, there is not much evidence for success in this type of approach. Learning disabilities certainly must be considered a heterogeneous disorder. The differences among students with learning disabilities are, however, probably too complex to allow us to base treatment on the child's membership in one of a limited number of broadly defined subgroups.

This is not to imply, however, that the team cannot learn much about the nature of the child's learning disabilities by examining test results and other data for specific patterns. After one has identified whether a learning disability exists, it may be helpful for those who are going to be working with the child to identify strengths and weaknesses in the child's learning style. In identifying strengths and weaknesses, the team should consider subtest patterns on the intelligence test as well as scores from some of the tests that were suggested as possible additions to the psychologist's battery. For example, it may be helpful for the child's teacher to know that he or she has excellent ability to perceive visual-spatial stimuli (as indicated by a high Performance IQ and good performance on a test of visual perception), but poor fine motor skills (as evidenced by slowness on the Coding subtest, sloppiness on the Mazes subtest, and poor performance on the Developmental Test of Visual-Motor Integration). The teacher then would know that he or she should not waste time on activities to strengthen visual-perceptual skills, but should instead work on strategies to remedy or circumvent the poor fine motor skills. Kaufman and Kaufman (1983) provide many suggestions for approaching children with various profiles on the K-ABC (difficulties with Simultaneous Processing, Sequential Processing, or both). Although strategies based on the test pattern profiles have reasonable face validity, there is little evidence that they are the most effective approaches to remediating the learning disabilities.

IDENTIFYING ASSOCIATED PROBLEMS

In addition to diagnosing learning disabilities and identifying areas of strength and weakness in the cognitive and achievement profiles, the team should attempt to identify associated problems that may be interfering with learning. Many of the problems that teachers consider most disruptive to the learning process are sometimes thought of as "behavior problems." By better understanding the basis of these problems, the teacher can better help the child overcome them. The interdisciplinary team has available several sources of data for identifying these problems that interfere with learning: teacher reports, parents reports, child interview, classroom observation, neurodevelopmental evaluation, test results, observation during testing, and subtest profiles. Various combinations of these data will be needed to identify the problems that exacerbate, or are exacerbated by, the learning disabilities.

Attention-Deficit Hyperactivity Disorder

A disorder commonly seen in conjunction with learning disabilities is attention-deficit hyperactivity disorder (ADHD). According to the Diagnostic and Statistical Manual of Mental Disorders, Third Edition-Revised ([DSM-III-R], American Psychiatric Association, 1987), for a child to be diagnosed as ADHD, he or she must meet criteria for developmentally inappropriate *inattention* (e.g., failure to finish things he or she starts, failure to listen, easy distractibility, difficulty in concentrating and/or sticking to a play activity), criteria for *impulsivity* (e.g., acting before thinking, shifting from one activity to another, difficulty in organization, need for supervision, frequent calling out in class, and difficulty awaiting turns), and criteria for *hyperactivity* (difficulty sitting still or staying seated, excessive running or climbing, fidgeting, and so on). A child with this disorder typically exhibits an inconsistent application of cognitive abilities to academic tasks, producing variable and inconsistent performance that confounds teachers, parents, and the child.

In the DSM III-R an attempt is made to distinguish between attention-deficit hyperactivity disorder (ADHD) and "undifferentiated attention-deficit disorder" (p. 52). This latter "residual category" is utilized to "describe disturbances in which the predominant feature is persistence of developmentally inappropriate and marked inattention that is not a symptom of another disorder, such as . . . attention-deficit hyperactivity disorder" (p. 95), and when signs of impulsivity and hyperactivity are not present. In the parlance of the Diagnostic and Statistical Manual of Mental Disorders-Third Edition ([DSM III], American Psychiatric Association, 1980), undifferentiated attention-deficit disorder would have been categorized as attention deficit disorder without hyperactivity. We feel that it is important to appreciate, both diagnostically and therapeutically, that disorders of attention and a physically high motor activity level may exist separately or together. Although it is rare, there are children who exhibit hyperactivity with no apparent attention deficits. More common are children with attention deficits with no apparent excesses of physical activity. The subclassification of ADHD within disruptive behavior disorders (subclass includes ADHD, oppositional defiant disorder, and conduct disorder) in the DSM III-R has the unfortunate consequence that deficits of attention span and excessive motor activity (hyperactivity) are made to seem the same, and the clinical and therapeutic needs for separation of these entities suffers. Again, as indicated in Chapter 1, to fall in concurrence with present diagnostic policy, we will, despite these misgivings, employ the term ADHD in subsequent discussion.

The diagnostic elements of ADHD are the finding of developmentally inappropriate attention deficits, poor impulse control, and exaggerated motor activity level. Although identification of attention deficits seems simple, it is sometimes a complicated process. It may be very difficult to determine whether a child's failure to perform stems from an attention span that is inappropriate for his or her cognitive level or whether there is an overall cognitive delay that would entitle a child to a degree of inattentiveness appropriate to the more immature level of functioning. Ascertaining correspondence between cognitive level and attention span is a bit simpler process for the child with substantial cognitive delays (e.g., mental retardation), but can be an extremely difficult process with children in a more normal range of function.

The interdisciplinary team needs to combine data from several sources to determine if ADHD is a problem associated with the learning disability. More emphasis should be placed on data gathered from the environment in which the child typically functions (i.e., the classroom and the home) than on data from the clinicians' evaluations, as the child may not display distractibility, impulsivity, and hyperactivity in the novel one-on-one situation.

The team will want to consider information gathered through the teacher'(s) interview, focusing especially on items regarding the child's activity level, ability to pay attention, follow directions, complete assignments, and control impulsivity. Similar information gathered through a classroom observation also should be considered. Data gathered from the parent interview will be of great importance in determining the existence of ADHD. The team should focus especially on the parents' responses to questions regarding the child's ability to listen to and follow directions, complete regular chores, and complete homework. Observations by the physician, psychologist, and educator who conducted testing with the child may provide important information in making the ADHD diagnosis. (See specifically Chapter 4 for discussion of some of the test behaviors that might indicate distractibility.)

Some of the most important diagnostic clues from the individual assessments (medicine, psychology, and special education) are discussed as follows:

Inattentiveness may be evident from the neurodevelopmental assessment in terms of variability in performance with tests of rote auditory memory, including, on occasion, an improved performance with digits reversed as opposed to digits forward, and in impulsive execution of the Gesell drawings (see Chapter 3).

In the medical, psychological, and special education assessments, a child with ADHD may evidence difficulty paying attention and staying on task, frequent requests for repetition of oral questions and directions, easy distractibility to visual and auditory stimuli, irrelevant comments or attempts to relate personal experiences that are brought to mind by various test stimuli, and tendencies to "lose track" of the tasks presented. The impulsive components of ADHD may manifest as tendencies to give the first answer that comes to mind, to begin tasks before instructions are completed, and to grab for materials before the examiner is ready to present them.

From the psychological assessment, a pattern of excessive distractibility can be hypothesized when relatively low scores are obtained on the WISC-R Arithmetic, Digit Span, and Coding subtests or on the K-ABC Magic Window, Face Recognition, Hand Movements, Number Recall, Word Order, and Spatial Memory. (See Chapter 4 for a discussion of subtest patterns.) These subtests, which are affected by the child's ability to focus attention, also are affected by many other unrelated factors. For this reason, a pattern of poor performance on these subtests should not be used as the primary determinant for making a diagnosis of ADHD. The team should use the subtest patterns in conjunction with some of the general observations listed previously to help identify ADHD.

To repeat, in the diagnosis of ADHD it is important to assess attention span within the setting in which the child is asked to function, that is, in the classroom. This assessment requires discussion with school personnel to determine the appropriateness of that situation and the child's attentional profile in the school setting with its attendant demands and distractions. It is inappropriate to attempt to diagnose ADHD without input from the school.

As stated previously, there is no single measure that can confirm or deny the existence of ADHD. Only by considering data from many sources can the diagnosis be made, and even then it is often difficult to be certain. Because the pertinent issue is the child's attention span, impulse control, and activity level in the home and school settings, professionals on the interdisciplinary team should place greater value on parents' and teachers' reports than on their own observations during evaluations of the child.

It is important to note here that ADHD sometimes is seen in children who are doing poorly in school but who do not exhibit learning disabilities. Many of these children have managed to master skills in basic academic areas (reading, mathematics, written language), but do poorly in school because they are unable to stay on task, complete assignments, and organize themselves. The strategies discussed in Chapter 10 for dealing with attention problems are equally appropriate for the child who exhibits ADHD with or without learning disabilities.

Problems with Organizational Skills or Study Skills

Children with ADHD often demonstrate difficulties with organizational and study skills. However, these problems can be observed in other children with learning problems as well and will, therefore, be discussed separately. As with the diagnosis of ADHD, the primary sources of data for identifying problems in organizational and study skills are the teachers, parents, and, if appropriate, the student. Their responses to questions regarding completion of homework (amount of homework assigned, actual time taken to complete it, need for supervision), reasons for poor grades (lack of preparation for tests, failure to complete homework or classwork, lack of class participation), and the child's need for structure at home and school will be important for determining if there are problems with organizational and study skills. Relevant information may also be gathered from observation of the child during testing and from the results of certain intelligence subtests that require good planning ability. (See Chapter 4 for a discussion of these subtests.) It is important to note that problems with organizational and study skills are observed more frequently as the child gets older and is expected to take more responsibility. Especially as children reach middle school, they often are expected for the first time to move from class to class on their own, and no longer have one primary teacher who will "look out" for them. Also, as children get older, long-term assignments are made that require more planning, more independent studying of texts is required, and parents often provide less supervision of homework.

Handwriting Slowness and Inefficiency

Although difficulties in written language usually are considered when making the diagnosis of learning disability, many of the tests that measure abilities in this area focus primarily on spelling and the mechanics of writing (e.g., punctuation, grammar, capitalization, word usage). Handwriting speed and efficiency, which is largely based on fine motor skill or visual-motor integration, is less often measured, but can play an important role in determining whether a child is able to perform in school at a level commensurate with his or her intellectual functioning. To determine if handwriting speed and efficiency are adequate, the interdisciplinary team should review data from the occupational therapy evaluation (if performed) and information from the teacher and parent interviews, focussing particularly on responses to questions regarding completion of assignments, time needed to complete assignments, and neatness of work. If possible, teachers should be questioned regarding the reasons for slow or inaccurate completion of assignments (e.g., daydreaming, slow but diligent work pace, failure to follow instructions, difficulty copying from the board).

Children with slow or inefficient handwriting often show difficulties with other fine motor skills, such as those presented during the occupational therapy evaluation or the neurodevelopmental evaluation. Scores on certain tests (e.g., tests of visual-motor integration, WISC-R Coding subtest) may be low. Observation during testing may also indicate reasons for the child's slow completion of assignments (e.g., perfectionistic approach, tendency to repeatedly lose his or her place during copying, off-task behaviors, awkward pencil grasp). Specific suggestions for circumventing handwriting difficulties can be made if the team can pinpoint the areas of weakness. (See Chapter 9 for a discussion of these strategies.)

Gross Motor Clumsiness

Some children with learning disabilities also demonstrate poor gross motor skills. These gross motor (play) skills represent one of the two major ways children relate to each other (the other being language). Although poor gross motor skills may not interfere with learning per se, they certainly can affect the already vulnerable self-concept of the child with learning disabilities. Difficulties with gross motor skills are assessed through the occupational therapy evaluation and the neurodevelopmental examination. Teachers and parents will often comment regarding a child's clumsiness. Responses to questions about extracurricular activities (especially athletics) will provide data regarding the extent to which gross motor difficulties influence the child's selection of pastimes.

Language or Speech Problems

Children with learning disabilities often have a history of slow language development. Language problems may continue into school age. Language problems may be mentioned first by parents or teachers, who might say that the child appears to have difficulty processing information, gives inappropriate responses to questions, has weak vocabulary skills, and is unable to relate common experiences or tell stories. Language difficulties also might be evidenced by a WISC-R profile where the PIQ is significantly and unusually higher than the VIQ. Observation during medical, psychological, and educational testing might also suggest language difficulties. (See Chapter 4 for a discussion of some of the signs examiners might observe in children with language difficulties.) A complete language evaluation should be obtained for children with suspected language difficulties. (See Chapter 6 for a discussion of the language evaluation.)

Speech problems will be observed more easily. The interdisciplinary team should attempt to determine whether speech difficulties are severe enough to interfere with learning. Consideration also should be given to the effects of speech difficulties on social/emotional adjustment. Evaluation by a speech pathologist will provide important information in determining the need for speech therapy.

Significant delays in speech or language warrant special education services, regardless of the existence of learning disabilities.

Emotional Problems

The child whose learning difficulties are assumed to be primarily the result of emotional handicaps is not diagnosed as learning disabled. However, the child with learning disabilities can and often does have concomitant secondary emotional difficulties. If learning disabilities are thought to be the primary handicapping condition, special education services that lead to improved academic achievement may be sufficient to correct emotional problems. Conversely, if an emotional disorder is the primary handicapping condition, psychotherapy may be sufficient to correct the learning problems. However, it is sometimes difficult to determine the primary handicapping condition—that is, to determine whether emotional problems are causing learning difficulties or vice versa. Regardless of the cause-effect relationship, the child with serious emotional and learning difficulties will benefit from help with both.

Data for determining the existence of emotional problems may come initially from the interview with the parents, teachers, and child. The team should focus especially on responses to questions regarding the child's self-concept, peer relations, eating or sleeping disorders, separation difficulties, level of motivation, unusual fears, mood swings, tendency to withdraw, and so forth. Observation during testing also will play an important role in identifying emotional disturbance. The child who shows excessive anxiety, anger, destructiveness, lack of confidence in his or her responses, avoidance behaviors, lack of eye-contact, inappropriate demonstrations of affection, low tolerance for frustration, or inappropriate affect should receive further evaluation. Results from projective psychological tests will be of value in making a determination regarding the presence of emotional disorders.

Family Problems

The presence of a child with learning disabilities, especially one who has associated ADHD, can be very disruptive to family life. Parents (and teachers) may feel the child is lazy, not working up to his or her potential, deliberately failing to follow instructions, stubborn and willful, or simply "dumb." Some parents may blame their child for poor school performance, rather than being supportive and attempting to help the child overcome his or her difficulties. Other parents may blame themselves for the child's difficulties and try to overcompensate by making excuses, providing excessive help with assignments, or allowing the child to avoid school. Especially as children get older, parents expect them to take more responsibility for their schoolwork, but become frustrated as they observe their child fail to do so. Children become more resentful of parental interference with school work, although they need the additional structure.

Identification of family problems is based primarily on information gathered from interview with the parent and the child. School personnel also may be aware of information pertinent to this topic. Projective tests also can provide valuable insights into family dynamics.

Specific Behavior Problems

Most behavior problems that will be mentioned by parents and teachers are, broadly speaking, manifestations of the child's reaction to his learning disability, ADHD, or emotional problems. Therefore, the strategies used to deal with these disabilities and disorders (e.g., special education services, medication, psychotherapy) generally will be effective in improving the child's overall behavior and in reducing specific behavior problems. Many specific behavior problems will, however, respond well to behavior management techniques (described in Chapter 11). It is, therefore, advisable to identify the most salient problems at home (e.g., lying, failure to follow instructions, difficulty getting ready for school, temper tantrums, excessive fighting with siblings) and at school (e.g., failure to complete assignments, talking out of turn, wandering about the classroom, tardiness). Interviews conducted with the parents and teachers are generally the best sources for identifying these problems. When possible, attempts should be made to identify the nature of the problem, when and where the problem is most likely to occur, any specific occurrences that are likely to trigger the problem, strategies that have been used in an attempt to control the problem, and the success of these strategies. Specific behavior management strategies can be suggested by the interdisciplinary team if this information is gathered carefully and clearly presented.

CONCLUSION

As outlined in this chapter, the first task of the interdisciplinary team, when it meets to review the individual team members' data, is to determine whether a significant discrepancy exists between the child's level of cognitive functioning and level of academic achievement in one or more areas. Appropriate and inappropriate methods for determining whether this discrepancy is significant were discussed. Because learning disabilities cannot be defined strictly according to statistical formulae, the team is urged to consider factors in addition to test performance. The next task is to examine data from a variety of sources to determine factors that underlie the disability or help to clarify its nature. Finally, the team must determine the existence of problems often associated with learning disabilities. After completing this procedure, the team will have the information necessary to develop a comprehensive plan for treatment.

PART II:

PLANNING FOR TREATMENT

CHAPTER 9

Planning for Treatment of Learning Disabilities and Associated Primary Handicapping Conditions

Elizabeth H. Aylward
Frank R. Brown, III
Winnie Dunn
Linda K. Elksnin
Nick Elksnin

Chapter 8 included discussion of the diagnosis of learning disabilities, ADHD, and associated problems. It is important for the team, once it begins to develop therapeutic recommendations, to appreciate that some of these conditions are neurologically based. The primary handicapping conditions include (but are not limited to) learning disabilities, speech-language disabilities, gross and fine motor difficulties, and ADHD. Because of these primary neurological handicapping conditions, the child with learning disabilities (if provided with no special programming) falls progressively behind in achievement, and may develop a variety of secondary handicapping conditions, including behavioral and emotional problems. Treatment of learning disabilities is the subject of this chapter. Treatment of ADHD will be discussed in Chapter 10. Treatment of secondary handicapping conditions will be discussed in Chapter 11.

In planning for treatment of the learning disabilities, team members must keep in mind that special education services are mandated in the Education for All Handicapped Children Act (Public Law 94-142). Public Law 94-142 requires the provision of a free, appropriate public education for all students identified as handicapped. Furthermore, it defines learning disability as a handicap, and requires that services for students with learning disabilities be provided in the least restrictive environment, that is, in a setting that permits the student with learning disabilities to remain among nonhandicapped peers as much as possible. The Education of the Handicapped Amendments (P. L. 99-457) provides new incentives for the development of services to preschoolers who are handicapped and their families.

As outlined in Chapter 1, the interdisciplinary team will diagnose primary and secondary handicapping conditions and develop general therapeutic recommendations. For example, the team may recommend that a child with reading disability be provided with reading resource help and special accommodations to help circumvent reading difficulties in other subjects. The interdisciplinary team usually will not outline the specific goals and objectives to be accomplished as part of the child's curriculum for the school year or specify particular instructional methods. Individual team members will be given responsibility for ensuring that more specific guidelines are developed and implemented. The following sections discuss the development and implementation of a plan for providing the special education and related services that are legally mandated for the student with learning disabilities as well as the preschooler deemed to be at risk for subsequent learning difficulties.

THE INDIVIDUALIZED EDUCATIONAL PLAN (IEP) AND THE INDIVIDUALIZED FAMILY SERVICE PLAN (IFSP)

The Individualized Educational Plan (IEP), required by P. L. 94-142, is a comprehensive plan of instructional activities to meet the needs of the school-age child. The IEP specifies "child-centered" goals and objectives, as well as the strategies and timetables for reaching them. The Education of the Handicapped Amendments (Public Law 99-457) extends initiatives of P. L. 94-142 to infants, toddlers, preschoolers, and their families. Public Law 99-457 emphasizes a "family-centered" approach to intervention, as opposed to the more child-centered approach of the IEP. The Individualized Family Service Plan (IFSP) is the statement of these family centered goals and objectives, as well as the strategies for reaching them.

The IEP/IFSP Development Team

The IEP is developed by a committee, usually based in the child's school. This committee might be composed of the same members as the interdisciplinary team. In most cases, however, the IEP development committee will be composed primarily of school-based personnel, with selected input from outside professionals. The committee usually includes the child's current teacher, a special educator, a school psychologist, and an administrator. The committee sometimes will solicit the participation of other professionals, either from the school or community (e.g., physicians, speech-language therapists, behavioral psychologists, occupational and physical therapists). It is helpful if at least one member of the interdisciplinary team assists in developing the IEP or is at least readily available to the IEP development committee. In addition to professional staff, parents should be asked to contribute their understanding of their child's needs, as well as their desires for outcome.

The IFSP is developed from child and family assessments conducted by an interdisciplinary team, much as outlined above for the IEP. Public Law 99-457 emphasizes the importance of participation of families in design of programs for their child and family, and as such, this legislation stipulates that the IFSP must be developed with at least one of the child's parents or the child's guardian participating in the process. The goal in development of both the IFSP and IEP is that parents be offered an opportunity to contribute their understanding of their child's needs, as well as their desires for outcome. In both the IFSP and IEP, parents are helped to understand their child's developmental and learning strengths and weaknesses and are encouraged to assist in the development of reasonable and realistic goals for remediation and instruction.

Components of the IEP

Although, by definition, each IEP is individualized to meet the particular student's needs, all IEPs have certain components in common, including:

1. *Current Levels of Achievement* must be stated from the most recent assessments. Scores or levels should be stated in understand-

able terms, so that members of the IEP development committee (including parents) can comprehend them.

2. Planning for the student with learning disabilities should reflect *goals*, that is, the committees' expectations for the student's accomplishments in a particular area during the period specified. The committee must specify short-term *objectives* for attainment of the goal, that is, measurable or observable steps toward the achievement of the goal.

3. Appropriate objective *criteria* must be included to determine if and when an objective is achieved. Such criteria may be stated as a percentage or as a ratio. Criteria can change throughout the course of programming.

4. The IEP should indicate the extent of special education (*specific services*) and related services that will be needed to help the student meet the outlined goals and objectives. The amount of time the child will spend receiving special services often is defined according to levels. (These levels will be addressed later in the chapter.) Related services represent intervention provided by professionals other than educators and may include, for example, speech-language therapy, occupational therapy, physical therapy, or counseling. These services should be outlined, as well as the amount of time the child will need to spend with each specialist. In addition to specifying extent of specific services, the IEP may specify particular methods to be used with the student (specific remedial approaches will be elaborated later in this chapter.) The IEP may outline modifications to be made in the instructional program, such as special seating, special management techniques, supplemental equipment or materials, computer assistance, or cassette recorders to supplement note taking. Special remedial or treatment methods, such as sensory integration therapy, pragmatic language therapy, articulation therapy, supplementary vocational or prevocational training also may be specified.

5. An IEP should state when the program will take effect and when attainment of goals and objectives is expected (*duration*). Usually, duration is for either a school year (9 months) or a calendar year. An IEP can be reviewed, revised, or rewritten at any time during implementation (with the parents' knowledge and consent), but all IEPs must be reviewed and updated at least annually.

Components of the IFSP

Part H of P. L. 99-457 specifies the content of the IFSP and certain requirements for participation and implementation. According to Section 677(d), the IFSP must be a written document that contains the following:

1. A statement of the child's present levels of physical development, cognitive development, language and speech development, psychosocial development, and self-help skills, based on acceptable objective *criteria.*
2. A statement of the *family's strengths and needs* relating to enhancing the development of the family's infant who is handicapped.
3. A statement of major *outcomes* expected to be achieved for the child and family; the criteria, procedures, and timelines used to determine the degree to which progress toward the outcomes is being made, and whether revisions of the outcomes or services are necessary.
4. A statement of specific early intervention *services* necessary to meet the unique needs of the child and family, including the frequency, intensity, and method of delivering services.
5. Projected dates for initiation of services and the anticipated *duration* of the services.
6. The name of the case manager who will be responsible for implementing the plan and coordinating with other agencies and persons.
7. The steps to be taken to support the child's transition from early intervention into a preschool program.

IEPs and IFSPs should incorporate the components just outlined but should be designed to allow flexibility in their implementation. For example, several methods can be suggested in the IEP or IFSP for instruction of specific skills, criteria for attainment of objectives can be adjusted, and provisions can be made for allowing the child to demonstrate attainment of skills in a variety of ways (e.g., orally, in writing, with manipulation of objects).

Implementation of the IEP/IFSP

The IEP must be developed before a student is placed in special education programming, must be implemented no later than 30 days after its development, and must be reviewed 60 days after its implementation. The IEP development team periodically updates the IEP, noting objectives met, success of methods, and whether the IEP still reflects realistic programming. If the IEP is inappropriate in any area, it is revised. Change in the nature or level of services provided cannot be made without the parents' consent. An addendum to the IEP or an entirely new document can be drafted by the committee. The student remains in the current program until the modifications are approved.

The IEP must be reviewed 60 days after any major revisions. The IFSP must be reviewed at least once a year, and parents must receive a progress report on the IFSP every 6 months.

Considerations for Developing and Implementing the IEP

In developing and implementing the educational plan, consideration should be given to the following assumptions regarding the student with learning disabilities and the learning process.

Students with learning disabilities are "normal" people with special needs. Students with learning disabilities have the same desire to learn and the same desire for acceptance in the process as their peers. They are entitled to enjoy the learning process, to have a good self-concept, and to be able to relate as normally as possible to other children, despite their learning handicap. Without some accommodations in the learning process, they probably will not have these experiences.

Students with learning disabilities require more structure. Because children with learning disabilities often exhibit distractibility, poor impulse control, and poor organizational skills, they usually will benefit from increased structure and organization imposed from outside sources. Increased structure involves the clear presentation of expectations, clear delineation of consequences for meeting or failing to meet expectations, and consistency in feedback. Specific strategies for increasing structure and consistency are outlined in Chapter 10. Structure will also enhance the effectiveness of other treatment modalities (e.g., medication for ADHD, behavior management strategies).

Many students with learning disabilities require more control of distractions. Distractions in the classroom should be minimized to maximize the child's ability to attend. Suggestions for decreasing distractions are discussed in Chapter 10.

Students learn best through direct experience. Abstract concepts and prolonged debate of esoteric issues do not work well as a foundation for teaching the student with learning disabilities. Instruction should be practical, and teachers should ask themselves "What can the student do with what he or she is learning?" Topics of interest are generated from daily experiences, and, when possible, can be presented in conjunction with activities such as field trips, films, and special projects.

Skills taught in isolation have a transient effect. The curriculum for the child with learning disabilities should emphasize relationships among skills and repetition over time. Skills taught in one subject area should be reinforced in other subject areas. For example, application of language skills is not taught in the English or reading class alone, but must be reinforced by teachers in other content areas. Goals of today should relate to the goals of yesterday and tomorrow. The development of any curriculum for students with learning disabilities requires provision for repetition of concepts and procedures. Reinforcement and repetition will enhance internalization of concepts.

Learning is a multisensory experience. Internalization of concepts is believed to be enhanced though presentation in a variety of sensory modalities (e.g., visual, auditory, kinesthetic, and tactile). Multisensory strategies include audio-visual instruction, laboratory experiences, manipulation of materials, and so forth.

There is a point of diminishing return in remedial programming. In programming for the student with learning disabilities, there is sometimes an automatic assumption that more remediation is necessarily better. The goals of special education should include instruction in content as well as remediation of skills. For example, the fifth grader, who for remediation of word attack skills, is required to read first grade material, will not be provided with ideas, concepts, and information appropriate for his or her cognitive level. The child's vocabulary and fund of information will suffer as a result of "overremediation." There must, therefore, be an appropriate balance between remediation of skills and instruction in content. Of course, instruction in content will have to be modified to circumvent areas of weakness. Suggestions for such modifications (e.g., Talking Books) will be discussed later in this chapter.

The most important issue for the child with learning disabilities is how he or she feels about himself or herself. Well-balanced programming affords the student with learning disabilities an opportunity to shine in his or her areas of strength. Successful experiences will serve as a reminder that he or she is normal and capable, despite his or her handicapping condition. This reassurance will, in turn, encourage the child to use and develop his or her inherent strengths, thus enhancing self-concept.

If these opportunities for developing strengths are not provided, the reverse may occur. The child with a poor self-concept may realize less than his or her inherent potential, and the prospect of disability becomes self-fulfilling.

LEVELS OF SERVICE

Once a child has been identified as meeting the eligibility criteria for special education, the IEP details the extent and types of special education intervention required to enable the student to meet the goals and objectives. In determining the extent of special education required, the IEP development committee should keep in mind that P. L. 94-142 mandates education in the least restrictive environment. Depending on the nature and severity of the disability, placement in special education settings will vary along a continuum, extending from mildly intrusive modifications in instructional programming to complete exclusion from the mainstream of education. This continuum of special education services might be portrayed as in Figure 9-1 (Deno, 1973). As suggested by Figure 9-1, most children are placed in programs that offer the most normalized settings, such as regular classrooms and resource rooms. There will be fewer children requiring the more restrictive settings, such as self-contained classrooms and out-of-school placements.

Although the descriptive terms applied to each level of service and the number of levels may vary from state to state or from district to district, the concept of a continuum of available services generally is applied. The levels of service portrayed in Figure 9-1 will be described as follows:

Regular Classroom with Consultative Special Education Assistance to the Teacher. The regular classroom teacher may receive consultative assistance from professionals in a variety of areas (e.g., special education, psychology, speech-language therapy, occupational and physical therapy). At this level, there is no direct contact between these professionals and the student.

Regular Classroom with Limited Services Outside of Class. At this level of resource placement, the student typically receives up to an hour per day of instruction outside of the regular classroom. Resource help usually is restricted to one subject area. A resource teacher usually schedules three to four children at a time to work on similar specific skill deficits.

One difficulty with a resource room placement is that a child who may already have problems with distractibility, impulsivity, and organizational skills must now relate to two teachers and complete two separate sets of assignments. For this reason, it is essential for resource teachers and regular classroom teachers to have good communication and to coordinate assignments. Because the child typically must leave the regular class to receive resource help, it is important that the child not be held accountable for the regular class instruction he or she misses.

At this level, the child is receiving his or her first direct exposure to any type of special education service. Careful monitoring at this level is important to determine whether the special education services should be continued at the same level, expanded, or deleted. If the child's performance and behavior in the resource room is markedly

TREATMENT OF LD AND RELATED CONDITIONS

```
Regular Classroom with Consultative Special Education Assistance
                         to the Teacher
Regular Classroom with Limited Services Outside of Class
    (e.g., OT, PT, Resource Room, Speech-Language)
    Regular Classroom with Expanded Services
                   Outside of Class
       Self-Contained Special Education Class,
         with or without Outside Resources
              Out-of-School (Residential
                   or Day Setting)
```

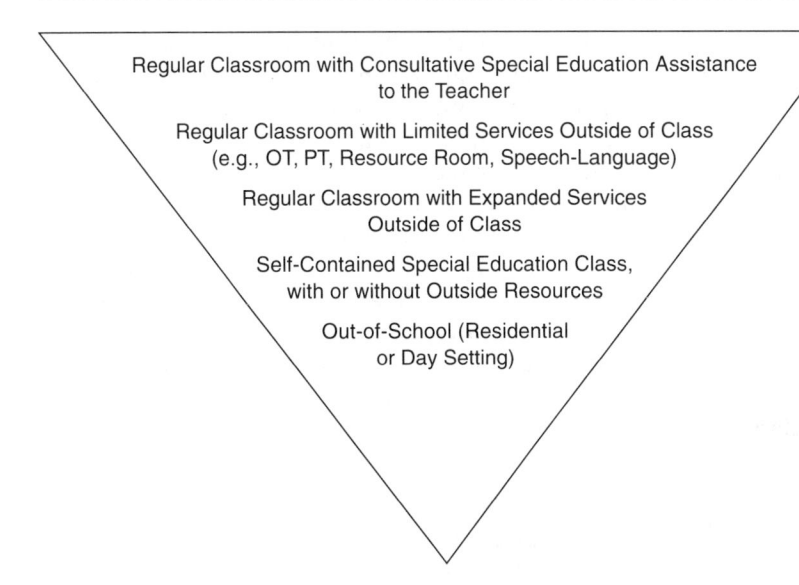

FIGURE 9-1. *Levels of Special Education Service*

better than his or her performance and behavior in the regular class, this may be a good indication that more resource help would be beneficial. In addition, the resource teacher is in a particularly good position to monitor the child's distractibility, impulsivity, and organizational skills, because the materials presented in the resource room are designed specifically to match the child's ability level and are presented in a less distracting environment.

Regular Classroom with Expanded Services Outside of Class. At this level of resource placement, the student typically spends up to one-half of each day (three hours) outside of the regular classroom. Resource help may be provided in more than one subject area. Considerations discussed in the previous paragraphs continue to apply at this level.

Self-Contained Special Education Class. If resource placement still is too distracting for the child, or if disabilities are too severe or too numerous, a self-contained classroom may be the best alternative. These classes usually contain 10 to 15 students with one special education teacher and perhaps an aide. Of course, a smaller pupil-teacher ratio is preferred. It is important that the student with learning disabilities be placed in a special education class designed specifically for students with similar learning disabilities.

In some schools, all children with learning difficulties are placed in noncategorical special education placements. Thus, slow learners, students with language deficits, and perhaps students who are retarded might be placed together with the students with learning disabilities. This is inappropriate and prevents the most efficient use of instructional time. Most school systems provide self-contained classrooms for a variety of disabling handicapping conditions, including mental retardation, orthopedic handicaps, communication disorders, emotional disturbances, and learning disabilities.

Out-of-School Placement. Out-of-school placements for children with learning disabilities generally are needed only for those students who have concomitant severe emotional or behavioral difficulties that prohibit their functioning in typical academic settings. Out-of-school placement also may be required in rural areas where there are too few students with learning disabilities to warrant special education classes within the school.

EDUCATIONAL APPROACHES TO REMEDIATE LEARNING DISABILITIES

In the section that follows, several instructional approaches that have been used effectively with students with learning disabilities will be reviewed. The first approach, Direct Instruction, is a model of instruction used to teach skills. The Strategies Intervention Model is an example of cognitive strategy instruction designed to teach students with learning disabilities *how* to learn rather than *what* to learn. Although academic instruction has received the bulk of attention of learning disabilities professionals, the need for social skills training has been recognized during the last decade, and this is the focus of the third model to be presented here.

Direct Instruction

Direct Instruction is an instructional model developed by Zigfried Engelmann and his colleagues at the University of Oregon. Successfully used with individuals with learning disabilities and other difficult-to-teach students, direct instruction has two major goals for students: skill mastery by every student and acquisition of skills at the fastest possible rate. This first goal is critical for students with learning disabilities. These students often become casualties of the general education curriculum as teachers move ahead even though students with learning disabilities failed to master critical grade-level objectives. It is equally important that students with learning disabilities be taught in the most efficient manner possible, as they generally lag behind their normally achieving peers in skill acquisition.

There are several distinctive features of the Direct Instructional (DI) model. Rather than use a loosely written lesson plan, the DI teacher presents a scripted teaching format, which is a series of steps carefully designed to effectively and efficiently teach a skill or concept. Although teachers may develop their own teaching formats, few teachers have the time for this activity and often rely on commercially available materials. *Reading Mastery* and *Corrective Reading* are examples of commercial DI reading instructional materials.

Direct Instruction usually occurs in small groups, depending upon the nature of the material and the age and ability of the student. Restricting group size permits the learning disabilities specialist to continually monitor student performance during oral and written lesson activities. Lower performing students are seated nearest the teacher to permit even more careful monitoring of their performance.

In a traditional classroom, the teacher asks a question, several students raise their hands, and one or two students are called upon to respond. Students with specific learning disabilities may rarely volunteer to answer a question or may be ridiculed by peers if they volunteer an incorrect answer. Students also may get the message that they can be passive learners in the classroom and cruise on "automatic pilot" after they have been called upon by the instructor. In DI lessons, 80% of responses are group responses. *Unison oral responding* permits the teacher to monitor student performance, allows every student in the group to participate in the learning process, and demands the attention of each student in the group.

Unison oral responding is achieved through the use of signals, or cues provided by the learning disabilities specialist. Teachers learn to use visual signals (e.g., pointing or touching to a stimulus) when students should be attending to the instructor or the instructor's material, and auditory signals (e.g., finger snaps, claps, and so on) when students' attention is directed toward their own materials.

The use of signals to elicit unison oral responding during small group instruction enables the teacher to monitor student performance and to correct incorrect responses. Errors are regarded as learning opportunities and each error is corrected in the group immediately and positively. Specific error correction procedures are used depending upon the type of error committed.

Direct Instruction lessons are presented at a rapid pace to sustain students' attention, minimize errors, and to reduce the amount of time wasted during instruction. The goal of a DI lesson is an average of nine student responses per minute. Results of studies designed to assess the efficacy of Direct Instruction are reported by Carnine (1979) and Gersten (1985), and the use of DI with students with disabilities in the regular classroom has been recommended by Larrivee (1989).

Cognitive Strategies Instruction

Students with learning disabilities often lack effective and efficient strategies for solving academic and social problems. For example, if you wanted to remember an unfamiliar phone number, you would begin by assessing your memory ability. You may decide that you need to write the number down on a piece of paper. If paper and pencil were unavailable, you would generate a strategy or strategies you could use to remember the information. You may rely on verbal rehearsal and repeat the number several times; you may cluster pieces of information and try to remember the first three numbers of the exchange (e.g., 792), and the next two numbers (52), and the last two numbers (19); you may remember a number by associating it with an important date (813-1492); or you may remember the number by visualizing the pattern the number makes on the touch-pad of the telephone. You would monitor and evaluate the use of your strategy and make modifications and adjustments if necessary. Many students with learning disabilities are unable to realistically assess their cognitive abilities; in addition they possess few effective strategies. Cognitive strategy instruction enables students with learning disabilities to become more efficient learners. Although several models of cognitive strategy instruction have been proposed (Pressley, 1990; Reid and Stone, 1991), the Strategies Intervention Model developed by Deshler and Schumaker and their colleagues at the University of Kansas Institute for Research in Learning Disabilities is implemented in many schools by learning disabilities professionals.

The Learning Strategies Curriculum of the Strategies Intervention Model is designed to teach students how to learn content material. In addition to giving the student with learning disabilities a series of steps that can be followed to take a test more efficiently, paraphrase, write a paragraph, and so forth, students learn *when* to use each strategy to promote generalization across settings and situations. Learning Strategies form three strands: acquisition, storage, and demonstration of competence. An example of an acquisition strand strategy is the Word Identification Strategy, which teaches students to decode unknown multisyllabic words. The First Letter Mnemonic Strategy helps students store information more efficiently through the generation of lists as memorization aids. Students with learning disabilities are able to demonstrate competence by learning the Error Monitoring Strategy, which they use to detect and correct errors in their written work.

Each learning strategy is taught using the same eight-step instructional process (Schumaker, Deshler, Alley, & Warner, 1983):

Step 1: Pretest and Obtain a Commitment to Learn. The student's current level of performance is determined. Areas of weakness are discussed with the student and the student is asked to commit to learning the learning strategy.

Step 2: Describe. During this step the teacher describes strategy steps, along with giving students reasons for using the strategy.

Step 3: Model. The teacher models each step in the strategy by "thinking out loud."

Step 4: Verbal Rehearsal. The teacher leads the group in "rapid-fire verbal rehearsal," which requires each student to say a step in the strategy using a round-robin format.

Step 5: Controlled Practice and Feedback. Because the teacher primarily is interested in strategy mastery, students practice the strategy using "easy" materials. For example, if students are learning the paraphrasing strategy, which requires them to state the main idea and supporting details in a paragraph, they first practice using materials written at their reading levels rather than at their grade placement level.

Step 6: Grade-Appropriate Practice and Feedback. After students are proficient in using the strategy with less demanding materials, they learn to apply the strategy to materials used in their content area classes (e.g., English, history, social studies, health, and so forth).

Step 7: Posttest and Obtain Commitment to Generalize. Students are asked to generalize the use of a newly acquired strategy when posttest results indicate mastery of the strategy.

Step 8: Generalization. Three phases comprise the generalization step. During the *orientation phase,* the teacher and students discuss situations in which the strategy might be used, along with environmental cues that indicate when to use the strategy. Students also are encouraged to adapt the strategy to meet the demands of the situation. The student uses the strategy in a variety of situations during the *activation phase.* For example, the student might be asked to use the paraphrasing strategy in a social studies class and to report back to the learning disabilities teacher. The teacher occasionally conducts a probe to ensure the student is proficient in strategy use during the *maintenance phase.*

Social Skills Training

Historically, the learning disabilities field was concerned with students' academic performance. More recently, learning disabilities professionals have recognized the importance of social skills and the fact that children with learning disabilities often lack social competence. Deficient social skills are associated with lack of peer acceptance, poor academic performance, and adult mental health difficulties. Deficient social skills may be due to a variety of factors, including lack of knowledge, lack of practice, lack of reinforcement, or problem behaviors (e.g., aggression, withdrawal) that may interfere with social skills acquisition or performance (Gresham, 1990).

Social skills are taught using modeling, role-play, performance feedback, and transfer of training. After a social skill is described by the teacher, the skill is modeled by a socially competent individual. Students then are given an opportunity to practice using a skill during role-play exercises. Performance feedback involves giving the student specific, informative feedback regarding the positive as well as the negative aspects of the role-play. Performance feedback may be provided by other participants in the training group as well as the teacher. Students have been taught social skills using direct instruction and cognitive strategies instructional models.

There are several commercially available social skills curricula. These programs can be characterized as "skills-specific" or as "problem-solving" approaches. A skills-specific program teaches discrete social skills: each skill is defined and task-analyzed to determine the skill steps. Problem-solving approaches teach students to identify a social or academic problem, generate potential solution strategies, implement a strategy, and evaluate outcomes. The most powerful social skills training program may involve both approaches, with the skills-specific approach enabling the student to expand his or her social skills repertoire, making it easier for the student to generate a wide array of solution strategies during problem-solving activities.

APPROACHES TO REMEDIATING PRIMARY HANDICAPPING CONDITIONS ASSOCIATED WITH LEARNING DISABILITIES

Speech-Language Therapy for Children with Learning Disabilities

The majority of children with learning disabilities and intercurrent language disabilities display relatively mild language disorders. Their school placement and intervention needs will differ from the smaller percentage of children with learning disabilities diagnosed as having more severe "communication disorders."

For those children diagnosed as having a mild language disorder in conjunction with a learning disability, assignment to a regular classroom with resource services provided by a certified speech-language pathologist will be appropriate. The speech-language pathology services will be designed to meet the individual child's need (based on information obtained through the language assessment) and they may include diagnostic therapy (extension testing), comprehensive direct clinical intervention, or a specific program designed in association with and delivered in part by other members of the interdisciplinary team (e.g., occupational therapy). Children assigned to such resource speech-language programs are not excluded from obtaining the benefits of consultation and support services provided to classroom teachers and families; rather, these benefits are recommended as additional services provided on an as-needed basis.

For the child with learning disabilities and more severe intercurrent language disability, it is the responsibility of the speech-language pathologist and the rest of the interdisciplinary team to determine whether the child's needs would be best met in a learning-disabled or a communication-disordered classroom. This decision will hinge in large part upon the team's perception of whether the child's major handicapping condition is the learning disability with an associated language deficit or vice versa. Additional factors might include whether it is anticipated that the child will require specially designed curriculum of the speech-language pathologist, and whether language disabilities are of severe enough degree to cause a child to significantly lag behind other children socially. If, on balance, the language disability is felt to be the predominant cause of disability, a decision may be made to place the child in a self-contained program for children with primary communication disorder (and the associated learning disabilities will be addressed within this classroom setting). Specific speech-language intervention methods and strategies will not be addressed here, rather the interested reader may refer to texts by Wiig and Semel (1984).

Occupational Therapy Program Implementation

After gathering information about the student's abilities and needs, and the supports and barriers in the environment, the occupational therapist creates interventions that make the best possible use of the individual's resources and the resources of the environment to optimize educational outcomes. Occupational therapists may address specific skills (e.g., handwriting) or the basic foundational skills requisite for performing academic tasks (e.g., postural control).

Occupational therapists employ several theoretical frameworks when addressing the needs of students with learning disabilities. One important framework, *sensory integration,* (Ayres 1972b, 1980), addresses the individual's sensory processing abilities, and the subsequent ability to use that sensory input to create and carry out an appropriate response. Sensory integrative theory is based on the following principles (Dunn, 1988, 1991a, 1991b):

1. An individual must receive and understand sensory input before an adaptive response can occur.
2. Controlled sensory input is used to evoke an adaptive response.
3. Adaptive responses increase sensory input and organization toward more complex forms of response.
4. Child-selected activities are more likely to sustain performance and improve organization.

Controversy exists about the utility of sensory integrative theory for developing appropriate interventions for students with learning disabilities. Proponents report that carefully designed sensory integrative procedures enable the child to establish functional patterns of responding to environmental stimuli. Clinical validity and some research data (e.g., Ayres, 1972a, 1972b, 1976, 1977; Ayres & Mailloux, 1981; Ayres & Tickle, 1980; Montgomery & Richter, 1977; Ottenbacher, 1982) exist for this point of view, but further research is needed. Opponents question the relationship between sensorimotor activities and learning (Arendt, MacLean, & Baumeister, 1988).

Additional theoretical frameworks used by occupational therapists when addressing needs of children with learning disabilities include: *functional/adaptation, developmental,* and *behavioral/cognitive.* The functional/adaptation framework enables the occupational therapist to consider the impact of specifically identified problems in performance of specific tasks. Adaptations evolve from attempts to match the individual's abilities and limitations with environmental features. Using the developmental framework, the therapist considers the typical evolution of skills and milestones and selects strategies that will enhance skill development. When cognitive and pyschosocial issues are present, the occupational therapist works collaboratively with other professionals, using a behavioral and cognitive theoretical framework.

Occupational therapists employ four primary approaches to service provision: remediation, compensation, promotion, and prevention (Dunn et al., 1989). *Remediation,* the most common approach, attempts to identify the problem areas and creates strategies that will "fix" them. Although many remediation strategies have been evaluated systematically, others appear to have clinical validity but need to be tested systematically through research. A *compensatory* approach also acknowledges the individual's areas of difficulty, but seeks to by-

TREATMENT OF LD AND RELATED CONDITIONS   163

pass the underlying deficit through knowledge of the child's capacities and modification of his or her environment. A *promotion* approach, frequently used in early intervention programs, seeks to optimize the development of an individual's skills and abilities through design and provision of an optimal environment. A *prevention* approach is used when the professionals recognize risk factors and work to keep them from interfering with the child's ongoing development. This approach is most useful before the child has demonstrated a delay or disability. The goal is to create environmental modifications that will prevent the development of behaviors that may interfere with future learning.

Occupational therapists often provide direct services to children with learning disabilities, but can also use monitoring (supervised therapy) and consultation. The occupational therapist is most apt to be called upon to provide *direct services* when sensorimotor systems are disrupted, and this disruption is interfering with the student's ability to perform functional tasks. Whenever possible, the occupational therapist incorporates intervention strategies into the student's routine, so that the routine can begin to cue the student to perform more functionally. For example, the occupational therapist could work on postural control in the student's desk (e.g., having the student reach to pick up a dropped pencil), so that when this occurs later in the day, the student can use those skills in an actual demand situation.

Sometimes physical therapists (PT) and adaptive physical educators (APE) collaborate on sensorimotor issues. The PT is more likely to focus on the motor control and capacity of the individual to perform the task (e.g., strength, trunk control); the APE is more likely to take a perceptual motor approach, which has a more established group activity program sequence, with drills and practice toward development of specific motor skills (Clark, Mailloux, & Parham, 1989).

Monitoring is a model of service provision in which the therapist supervises another person who carries out the activities on a regular basis. The occupational therapist identifies the problem areas, creates interventions and instructs another person in how to carry out the interventions safely. The therapist also meets with the person carrying on the activities on a regular basis to ensure that the activities are being carried out correctly, adapt the activities as the child improves, and determine when the intervention can be discontinued or changed. This model provides ongoing support for the classroom routines and the teachers who see the students each day. Occupational therapists also use monitoring to assist parents when self-care and home skills are a problem.

In a *consultative model*, the occupational therapist addresses the needs identified by another individual in the student's environment (e.g., teacher, another therapist, physician, parent). A collaborative model of consultation is preferred because all parties contribute to problem identification and solutions (Idol, Paolucci-Whitcomb, & Nevin, 1986). A wide range of activities can occur within the collaborative consultation model, including adapting tasks, materials and environments, teaching adults new skills, and addressing postural and sensorimotor demands within natural environments.

Some students with learning disabilities receive services both from a school-based therapist and an occupational therapist in private practice. This situation occurs when the student has needs that extend beyond the educationally relevant needs the student demonstrates at school. Many of the problems that students with learning disabilities have also affect life at home and in the community, so this is an appropriate pattern of service provision. For example, the perceptual problems that interfere with the student's ability to get his answer on the right place on the page, can also interfere with his ability to tie his shoes or find clothes in the drawer. When both a school-based occupational therapist and a private practice therapist are serving a child, they collaborate to provide complementary services.

In all this service provision, it is important to recognize that individuals are best served when they are developing skills that are useful within naturally occurring activities throughout the day. Providing isolated services outside of the individual's routine does not address the need for those skills to generalize into the individual's life. Occupational therapists are particularly well suited to address the needs of individuals within their natural environments.

ACCOMMODATIONS TO CIRCUMVENT LEARNING DISABILITIES

As discussed previously, there must be a balance between amount of time spent in attempting to remediate weaknesses and amount of time spent in instruction of content. The student who is learning disabled, whose intelligence generally is average or above, must continue to be exposed to appropriate cognitive stimulation, despite the fact that academic skills are impaired. In order to provide this stimulation, teachers will have to make certain accommodations in their instructional methods, assignments, and methods of evaluation. The following paragraphs provide some suggestions on specific accommodations that may be necessary to ensure that the student who is learning disabled can fully utilize his or her cognitive potential and to ensure that his or her mastery of material is acknowledged.

Accommodations for Reading Disabilities

For the student with reading disabilities, it will be necessary to select (or develop) text material that presents content at the appropriate cognitive level, but that is written at the appropriate reading level. For students with less severe reading disabilities, the teacher may wish instead to read the regular text material together with the student, writing in appropriate substitutions for those words the student cannot decode alone.

Another approach, which allows the student to participate in regular classes and use regular text material, requires that the text material be dictated onto tape. This can be done by the teacher, parent, or another student. The student who is learning disabled then can listen to the tapes as he or she follows along in the text. Although time consuming for both teacher and student, this approach reinforces reading skills, while at the same time circumventing reading disabilities.

Parents and teachers should be aware that the U. S. Library of Congress provides a service known as Talking Books to individuals who are blind, reading disabled, or otherwise unable to read regular materials. Students who have documented reading disabilities can borrow, free of charge, tape-recorded versions of books and magazines, as well as a cassette tape player. Librarians at the school or public library should have information regarding this service. If not, parents or teachers should contact the Chief, Network Division, National Library Service for the Blind and Physically Handicapped, Library of Congress, Washington, D.C., 20542.

Students with reading disability also may need special accommodation in evaluation. For example, students may need to have someone read test items and test instructions to them. Extra time also might be allowed for completion of tests.

Accommodations for Mathematics Disability

Accommodations for children with learning disabilities in mathematics will depend upon the areas of specific weakness. If, for example, the child has difficulty with computation, but not mathematical concepts, he or she might be allowed to use a calculator when working on applied problems. Alternatively, he or she might be evaluated separately on his or her ability to determine the correct procedure for solving the problem and his or her ability to complete the calculations correctly. Some students may have difficulty remembering the sequence of steps needed for certain mathematical operations (e.g., long division, finding lowest common denominators) or may be distracted easily before completing all the steps. These students should be allowed to refer to a written list of steps for each problem. Children with handwriting difficulties often have trouble copying math problems. Accommodations should be made to avoid unnecessary copying. Of course, children with learning disabilities in math should be given extra time for tests.

Accommodations for Written Language Disability

Students with written language disability often demonstrate extreme frustration because they are unable to express their thoughts in writing. Despite the fact that they can gather information with no difficulty and process the information intelligently, their efforts often fail to be acknowledged because they are unable to demonstrate what they know in writing. Teachers should allow these students to substitute oral presentations for written assignments and to substitute oral tests for written tests. Whenever possible, tests should use an objective format (e.g., true/false, multiple choice) rather than an essay format. When written work is required in content areas, it should be evaluated on the basis of content, not spelling, mechanics, or organization. Alternatively, teachers might give one grade for content and one grade for writing.

Students whose written language difficulties are limited to the area of spelling might be encouraged to keep a list of those words that regularly give them trouble and be allowed to consult the list whenever necessary. These students might also benefit from the use of a word processor that automatically will check their work for spelling errors, or a hand-held spell checker.

Accommodations for Handwriting Difficulties

Because handwriting difficulties, like attention deficits, often are neurologically based, attempts at remediation in this area often are futile. For this reason, accommodations for students with poor or inefficient handwriting must be made to prevent excessive frustration. The suggestions made for accommodation of children with written language disability are equally appropriate for children with handwriting difficulties. In addition, the amount of written work required of these students should be decreased. Students with handwriting difficulties should be allowed to dictate assignments onto tape, or to dictate them to a parent or to another student. They should be allowed to use a tape recorder in class to supplement note-taking. If copying assignments from the blackboard presents problems, the student with handwriting difficulties should be allowed to dictate onto tape the material he or she does not have time to copy. Alternatively, another student might be asked to make a carbon copy when he or she is writing the assignment. Unnecessary copying should be avoided. For example, if an assignment requires students to copy sentences and underline the subject of each sentence, students with handwriting difficulties should be allowed to write only the subject of the sentence. These students may find it easier to use a typewriter or word processor than to write by hand (although poor fine motor skills often interfere with attempts to learn to type). If the student can learn to use a typewriter or word processor efficiently, he or she should be allowed to use it for both class assignments and homework.

CONCLUSION

After the interdisciplinary team has formulated diagnoses and outlined general recommendations for treating the disorders identified, a separate committee usually is convened to outline specific methods for remediating and circumventing learning disabilities. The Individualized Educational Plan (IEP) or Individualized Family Service Plan (IFSP) is written to outline the goals and objectives to be met during a specified period of time. The amount and type of special education services, related services, or family services that will be needed to help the child meet these goals are also outlined in the IEP or IFSP. Special instructional techniques, as well as accommodations needed to help the student circumvent weakness, must also be delineated. In developing and implementing the IEP or IFSP, the development committee must keep in mind that the most important component in the process is the child and the family. By pinpointing specific weaknesses, identifying potential strengths, and placing primary emphasis on the child's self-concept, the committee will be able to develop a plan that allows the child to meet the goals and objectives they have outlined, as well as to minimize the stigma of being labeled as "learning disabled."

CHAPTER 10

Planning for Treatment of Attention-Deficit Hyperactivity Disorder

Frank R. Brown, III
Elizabeth H. Aylward

In earlier chapters, we introduced a distinction between primary and secondary handicapping conditions for children with learning disabilities. As discussed, primary handicapping conditions are neurologically based, and include learning disabilities, speech-language disabilities, gross and fine motor dyscoordination, and attention-deficit hyperactivity disorder (ADHD). Chapter 9 discussed remediation of learning disabilities and any associated deficits in speech-language and gross or fine motor dyscoordination. This chapter addresses remediation of ADHD.

PLANNING FOR REMEDIATION OF ATTENTION-DEFICIT HYPERACTIVITY DISORDER

In general, children with learning disabilities exhibit two problems that might be associated with the word *attention*. They may have *too little attention* (span) and *too much attention* (seeking). The lack of a developmentally appropriate attention span (ADHD) represents a primary, neurologically based handicapping condition (analogous to learning disability) that is, for the most part, out of the child's control. This neurological deficit interferes with the learning process and compounds the already complicated learning disabilities profile. Attention seeking, on the other hand, is a secondary handicapping condition that is behaviorally rather than neurologically based and stems in part from the fact that children with learning disabilities do not receive the normal positive reinforcements that go along with school achievement. In reaction to this situation, the child with learning disabilities may exhibit a variety of negative attention-seeking behaviors that again interfere with the learning process.

The child with learning disabilities typically will exhibit some mixture of "attentional" problems, that is, both a lack of and an inordinate seeking of attention. This fact has created a lot of confusion in choosing appropriate environmental accommodations (both at home and at school), use of stimulant medications (e.g., methylphenidate, Ritalin), and behavior modification techniques. In this section, the two major treatment modalities for children with a primary attention deficit, environmental accommodations and stimulant medication, will be discussed. Chapter 11 will address behavior management strategies appropriate for children with secondary attention-seeking behaviors.

MANAGEMENT OF ATTENTION-DEFICIT HYPERACTIVITY DISORDER—ENVIRONMENTAL ACCOMMODATIONS

All children need structure and consistency. As children grow older, however, parents and teachers usually expect them to take more responsibility for their actions, to require less structure and supervision, and to be able to deal with less consistency in the daily routine. Children with primary neurologically based ADHD (who are often thought of as "immature") need more structure and consistency for a longer time than most children their age.

It is not easy, for many reasons, to deal with children who have ADHD. At times, they appear quite able to function at an age-appropriate level, making parents and teachers believe that the child's inappropriate behavior is completely volitional. At times (especially as they reach adolescence), children often resent interference from parents and teachers, and want to be responsible for themselves, but do not have the organizational abilities that will allow them to do so successfully. Their impulsivity causes them to do "stupid" things that they know are inappropriate, causing frustration for both themselves and adults.

Parents and teachers need to understand that ADHD is a primary, neurologically based disability that prevents children from paying attention, following instructions, organizing themselves and their materials, completing work on their own, tuning out distractions, and controlling impulsivity. Just as parents and teachers of a child who is physically impaired would not insist on taking away the child's wheelchair or braces when he or she reaches a certain age, parents and teachers should not insist that the child with ADHD function without the extra support, structure, and consistency he or she needs.

Parents and teachers will need to provide extra support, structure, and consistency of the type discussed in the remainder of this chapter to help the child with ADHD function. In some instances, these accommodations may be all that is required and they may obviate the need for stimulant medication. In most circumstances, however, one finds that environmental and behavioral accommodations, combined with administration of stimulant medication is more effective than any of these modalities by itself in minimizing the negative effects of ADHD.

School-Based Accommodations to Increase Structure and Consistency

Teachers of children with ADHD will have to make special efforts to provide the extra support and structure these children need, as well as attempting, as much as possible, to cut down on the number of distractions in the classroom. The following suggestions might be shared with the teachers of children who are diagnosed as having ADHD.

Children with ADHD have difficulty in making transitions from one activity to another. It is important, therefore, to keep the daily routine as consistent as possible. The child should be able to expect that various activities (e.g., reading, recess, lunch, physical education) will occur at approximately the same time each day. Changes from room to room and from teacher to teacher should be minimized, as the child often has difficulty making transitions and organizing himself or herself in new situations. If the child must be taken out of the room for special education services, the services should be provided at the same time every day. The child should not, of course, be expected to make up work he or she misses when taken out of the room for special education services. The special education services should be provided at the same time that the children in the regular class are being presented with material in the same subject area (e.g., special reading help should be provided at the same time as the regular class is having the reading lesson).

A child with ADHD will have more difficulty paying attention to classroom instruction. To work around this difficulty, teachers should make certain they have the child's attention before beginning instruction. This can be best accomplished by working with the child one-on-one or in a small group. Because this usually is impossible, teachers can use other strategies, such as standing next to the child, placing a hand on the child's shoulder, maintaining eye contact, and frequently asking direct questions to make certain the student is following along. When giving directions for a particular assignment, it may be necessary sometimes to repeat instructions individually for the child, or to ask him or her to repeat the instructions to make certain that he or she understands what is expected.

Directions for specific tasks or assignments should be stated precisely and simply. Young children should only be given one direction at a time. Older children may be able to remember two or three directions, but if the directions are at all complex, they should be put in writing. Teachers must specify clearly what they expect. For example, teachers should not ask the child with ADHD to "Organize your materials to go home." Instead, the child should be told to "Check to make certain you have your math book, homework assignment, and notebook."

The child with ADHD often becomes overwhelmed when faced with a large assignment. Teachers can help overcome this obstacle by breaking down tasks into small, manageable segments. For example, if the child has a page of 50 math problems to complete, the teacher should cover up 40 of them and tell the child only to complete the first 10 problems. After the first 10 are completed, verbal praise should be provided, and the next 10 problems should be uncovered. This procedure should be continued until all 50 problems are complete. Gradually, the child can be taught to break assignments into segments on his or her own and to provide his or her own verbal reinforcement.

It may be beneficial also to set a reasonable time limit for completion of each task. A kitchen timer will be helpful, as the child may not have a good concept of how much time is passing. Using the previous example, the teacher might tell the child he has 10 minutes to complete the first 10 problems. The teacher then should set the timer and come back when it rings. The child should be reinforced for completion of the segment, and the process repeated. The time limits can be adjusted as appropriate.

Teachers should attempt, as much as possible, to cut down on the number of distractions for the child with ADHD. Whenever possible, instruction should be provided individually or in small group settings. When instruction is provided in large group settings, the child should be seated near the teacher. When independent work is required, the child might benefit from the use of a study carrel. Alternatively, the child might be allowed to go to the library or other quiet place that would be relatively free of distractions. These strategies should only be used if they can be done in such a way that the child does not feel he or she is being punished by the isolation (for the obvious reason of the child's self-concept).

The classroom environment also may need to be modified for the child with ADHD. Too many posters, bulletin boards, and equipment will add unnecessary distraction. An "open space" environment is especially inappropriate because it prevents the teacher from controlling external auditory and visual distractions.

Teachers should attempt to provide plenty of reinforcement for successful completion of tasks. Verbal praise should be provided whenever there is improvement in the child's ability to complete tasks, work independently, or pay attention. Teachers should not expect major changes to happen quickly. By reinforcing the small gains, teachers can motivate the child to work toward larger gains.

These suggestions are for increasing structure and consistency for the child with ADHD. If there are specific behaviors that need improvement, teachers should be encouraged to establish a behavior management system, which will be described in Chapter 11.

Home-Based Accommodations to Increase Structure and Consistency

Some parents will need assistance from the professional team in providing the extra support, structure, and consistency their child needs. Depending upon the parents' level of sophistication, willingness to cooperate, and own level of organization, they may or may not need assistance in implementing the following strategies. The interdisciplinary team should not assume, however, that parents will be able to follow through in establishing effective behavior management strategies on their own. Regular follow-up will be needed to assist parents with this task. (See Chapter 13 for a discussion of follow-up with the families of children with learning disabilities).

The interdisciplinary team may want to share with the child's parents the following suggestions for home management of children with ADHD.

Parents should attempt to increase the structure of the daily routine. Children with ADHD have difficulty making transitions from one activity to another. It is important, therefore, to keep the daily routine as consistent as possible. Parents should try, as much as possible, to have the child do daily tasks—such as getting up in the morning, getting ready for school, eating meals, starting homework, getting ready for bed, bedtime—at the same time every day. As much as possible, the child should be allowed to finish each task before being asked to start another. For example, parents should not set up the daily schedule so that breakfast comes in the middle of getting ready for school.

A child with ADHD will have more difficulty in paying attention to directions. To work around this difficulty, parents should make certain they have the child's attention before giving instructions. For example, parents should not walk through the den and say "Pick up your shoes" while the child is watching television if they really expect the job to be done. Instead, the parent should first cut down all distractions as much as possible (turn the television off or get the child away from his or her friends or toys for a moment). The child should be called by name, and the parent should wait for a verbal response and eye contact. Instructions should be stated clearly and simply. Younger children should be given only one instruction at a time. Older children may be able to remember two or more directions, but if the directions are at all complex, they will need to be put in writing. The child might be asked to repeat the instructions so the parent knows the child understands what is expected.

When giving instructions parents should specify clearly what they expect. For example, the child with ADHD should not be told to "clean your room." Instead, parents should indicate specifically what they mean by "clean your room." (The parent's idea of a clean room and the child's idea of a clean room are probably not the same.) Parents might, for example, say instead, "Pick up your clothes. Put the dirty ones in the hamper. Hang up the clean clothes. Put toys in the toy chest. Empty your waste basket. Make your bed." (Instructions, should not, however, be presented all at one time. Parents may need to give each instruction separately and check to see whether the child has carried it out before giving the next instruction, or instructions might be put in writing.)

The child with ADHD often becomes overwhelmed when faced with a large assignment. Parents can help the child overcome this obstacle by breaking down tasks into small, manageable segments. For example, if the child has difficulty getting himself ready for school, the parent might divide the task into segments by first asking the child to wash his or her hands and face. After this is done, the parent should provide verbal praise and tell the child to get dressed. This procedure can be continued until all steps of the larger task have been completed. Gradually, the child can be taught to break tasks into segments without help and to provide his or her own verbal reinforcement.

It also may be beneficial to set a reasonable time limit for completion of each segment of a task. A kitchen timer will be helpful for the child who does not have a good concept of how much time has passed. The timer can be set, and the parent can come back when the timer rings. The child should be reinforced for completion of the segment and the process repeated. Time limits should be adjusted as appropriate.

If the task assigned is one that requires any amount of concentration, parents should attempt to cut down on the number of distractions as much as possible. Homework should not be completed in front of the television or in a room full of activity. Telephone calls should not be allowed during homework time. Some children complete homework best if sent to their room to work alone, but it is important to remember that even a quiet room may have lots of distractions, such as toys and books. It may be more convenient for parents to provide the supervision needed by having the child sit at the kitchen table or other centralized place, assuming that the area can be kept fairly quiet. Parents will need to experiment to see what works best for them and their child.

Parents should provide lots of reinforcement for successful completion of tasks. It is unreasonable to expect behaviors to change in one day. Parents must keep in mind how long it took the child to develop the bad habits they are attempting to correct, and realize that the resolution of these problems also may entail a great deal of time. Praise should be provided whenever improvement is observed, no matter how slight that improvement is. Parents should be encouraged to be patient and not give up.

Although the previous suggestions are based on psychological principles that have been tested and proven over the years, there always are exceptions to every rule. It is important for parents to remember that the list contains suggestions for helping their child work around attention problems, not steadfast rules. The suggestions should be implemented consistently for a few weeks. If something is not working, parents should experiment on their own to see if they can find a better approach.

These suggestions are for the management of general behaviors. If there are specific behaviors that need improvement, parents should be encouraged to establish a behavior management system, as described in Chapter 11.

MANAGEMENT OF ATTENTION-DEFICIT HYPERACTIVITY DISORDER—USE OF PSYCHOTROPIC MEDICATION

Approximately 50 years ago, a chance observation was made that stimulant medications (amphetamines) improved school performance and behavior and had a paradoxical calming effect on hyperactivity (Bradley, 1937). The use of stimulant medications proliferated, until by the late 1960s about 10 percent of children attending public schools were taking them. In the 1980s, however about

1.5 percent of children in the Baltimore school system received stimulant medications. The current decreased utilization of these medications reflects their earlier widespread misuse. Specifically, they frequently were used as a first recourse rather than as a component of a comprehensive remediation program (including environmental accommodations and behavioral modifications). They frequently were used as a "cure-all," which delayed implementation of more appropriate and specific interventions, and commonly, no monitoring systems were in place to assess their efficacy and needs for continuance. Secondary to these abuses, usage of stimulant medication has decreased to a point where it may, if anything, be currently underutilized.

Institution of psychotropic medication can be considered for any child who exhibits symptomatology compatible with ADHD, but only after evaluation of cognitive potential, academic achievement level, and assessment of the appropriateness of the existing academic placement. It should be remembered that medication is only one part of the management program for the child with ADHD. All team members participating in management of the child with learning disabilities and attention-deficit hyperactivity disorder will need to ensure that other important treatment modalities are not ignored.

Although other psychotropic medications have proven to have efficacy for children with ADHD, stimulant medications (methylphenidate hydrochloride [Ritalin], dextroamphetamine [Dexedrine], and pemoline [Cylert]) continue to be the medications of choice, because of demonstrated improved reaction time and accuracy (Rapoport, Zametkin, Donnelly, & Ismond, 1985) and because they seem to cause fewer and less serious side effects. It is our opinion that methylphenidate is the stimulant medication of choice for children with ADHD, and that related central nervous system stimulants (i.e., dextroamphetamine and pemoline) have no particular pharmacologic advantage over methylphenidate. We believe the physician should learn to use one of these medications effectively, and therefore in this discussion methylphenidate will be used as a prototype.

It is important to appreciate that, both diagnostically and therapeutically, disorders of attention (ADHD) and physical over-activity (hyperactivity) may exist separately or together. A number of studies point out that acute control of excessive motor activity (hyperactivity) with methylphenidate does not necessarily ensure academic improvement. In general, as the dosage of methylphenidate is raised, a child will become quieter. However, above a certain dosage (around 1.0 mg/kg/dose), the child's academic performance may start to decrease, even though he or she is physically less motorically active. A dosage of methylphenidate of approximately 0.3 to 0.6 mg/kg/dose generally is better for improving attention span, decreasing impulsivity, and maximizing reaction time, although it may not always reduce motor activity level (Sebrechts et al., 1986). Our recommendation is that a dosage of approximately 0.3 to 0.4 mg/kg/dose be used as a guideline for initiation of methylphenidate, and that this dosage be adjusted subsequently (up to a maximum of approximately 0.6 mg/kg/dose) on an individual basis. Parents should be alerted to anticipated initial mild side effects, consisting chiefly of loss of appetite and disturbance of sleep, as well as to the more serious side effect of an increase in frequency of tics in a child with underlying complex tic disorder (Tourette's syndrome). Loss of appetite and sleep disturbance can be minimized by starting with a low dosage (perhaps one-half of the anticipated optimal dosage) and increasing gradually for the first week or two to the optimal level (the smallest effective dosage).

The short-term benefits of stimulant medication are easily demonstrated and may include improvement in attention span and in relationships with peers, improvement on visual-motor tasks (handwriting), and decreased impulsiveness. Stimulant medication should be initiated on an empirical basis and should be continued based on feedback from the parents and school regarding its effects on attention span and impulse control. In this feedback process it is important to apprise parents and school personnel of what stimulant medication can and cannot do.

The desired effect is an improvement in attention span and impulse control, that is, the components of primary, neurologically based ADHD. Stimulant medication will not have an impact on behavioral problems under the child's willful control, such as oppositionalism, noncompliance, and attention-seeking. Because problems of ADHD (not under willful control, but affected by stimulant medication) and attention-seeking behaviors (under willful control, and not affected by stimulant medication) often occur together in children with learning disabilities, it is requisite that parents and school personnel be aware of what specifically to monitor when stimulant medication is employed. If they are not, they may erroneously conclude that medication has not helped (with willful behavior problems) and it may be discontinued prematurely.

The other responsibilities in monitoring stimulant medication usage are to know about its rate of metabolism, dosage adjustment, and when to discontinue it. Methylphenidate has a very short half-life in the blood stream of approximately 3 to 4 hours. This has several important ramifications for its administration:

1. Children will typically require two doses (approximately 8 A.M. and noontime) to cover the typical school day. If they are having

attentional interference with homework activities, they may require a third dose in the day, typically around 4 P.M.

2. Because of the rapid rate of metabolism, one is not concerned with the total dose administered in 24 hours, but rather with what is the correct individual dosage at any one time. This means that if the correct dosage at any one time is, for example, 10 mg, then this same dosage should be used at other times of administration in the day. One does not reduce subsequent dosages out of concern for the cumulative amount taken in the day.

3. A dosage of 0.3 to 0.4 mg/kg/dose is only a rough guideline (which implies that the typical school-age child will be taking approximately 10 mg/dose) and the dosage will have to be adjusted to fit each child. One usually starts with a somewhat lower dosage (e.g., 5 mg) and slowly increases the dosage to obtain the desired improvement in attention span and impulse control.

4. It now appears that a significant number of young children with ADHD will continue to exhibit symptoms, especially excessive fidgeting and restlessness (as opposed to gross motor overactivity), into adolescence and adulthood. The best way to monitor ongoing need for stimulant medication is to give the child drug vacations once or twice a year, monitoring attention span and impulse control before and after these drug interruptions. To remove day-to-day variations in performance, except in very obvious situations, these trials should be of approximately one to two weeks duration. If needs for continuance are monitored in this fashion, legitimate objections about open-ended medication usage can be obviated.

For those children with ADHD who show no therapeutic response to an adequate trial of methylphenidate, some alternative or adjunctive medications can be considered, especially the tricyclic antidepressants, imipramine (Tofranil) and desipramine (Norpramin), and the antihypertensive agent, clonidine hydrochloride (Catapres). Imipramine and desipramine have demonstrated value in the treatment of children with ADHD, especially in that subset with associated depressed mood and/or conduct disorder (Donnelly et al., 1986). The recommended dosage for imipramine is 0.5 to 3.0 mg/kg/day in 1 to 2 divided doses, and of desipramine, 2 to 4 mg/kg/day as a single dose. Clonidine hydrochloride can be useful, either as a sole agent, or in combination with methylphenidate. The recommended dosage is 0.03 μg/kg/day. The primary side effects of imipramine and desipramine are dry mouth, constipation, urinary retention, as well as disorders of coordination and movement, and of clonidine are hypotension, dry mouth, and drowsiness. Because the tricyclic antidepressants and clonidine have more significant side effects than the stimulant medications, they should not be used as a first line medication in the treatment of ADHD.

CONCLUSION

Learning disabilities and ADHD represent primary, neurologically based handicapping conditions, which are in large part beyond the child's control. Chapters 9 and 10 have addressed remediation of these primary handicapping conditions. It can be argued that separation of problems for the child with learning disabilities into primary handicapping conditions (e.g., learning disability and ADHD) and secondary handicapping conditions (e.g., attention-seeking behaviors and poor self-concept) is artificial, in the sense that a child with learning disabilities often has a mixture of these problems. Nevertheless, we feel that it is useful when thinking about remediation to separate initially the child's problems into those that are neurologically based (and beyond the child's control) and those that are more emotionally and behaviorally based.

The first step in addressing the needs of a child with learning disabilities will be to identify a remediation setting (as discussed in Chapter 9) that can provide an individualized educational course appropriate for the child's cognitive and academic strengths and weaknesses. The second step is to ensure that appropriate home-based and school-based accommodations are in place to help the child focus attention and control impulsivity. If the child continues to show attention deficits and poor impulse control, additional therapies, including stimulant medication (methylphenidate, Ritalin) can be instituted. Even when an individualized educational plan is established and primary ADHD is addressed in this fashion, many children with learning disabilities will be left with some secondary handicaps (e.g., attention-seeking behaviors and poor self-concept). Suggestions for minimizing these problems will be discussed in the following chapter.

CHAPTER 11

Planning for Treatment of Secondary Handicapping Conditions

Elizabeth H. Aylward
Frank R. Brown, III

The primary handicapping conditions of the child with learning disabilities (learning disabilities, speech-language disabilities, fine motor dyscoordination, and ADHD) are, as discussed in Chapters 9 and 10, "part of the child's wiring" and are, as such, somewhat out of his or her control. The strategies discussed for dealing with these primary handicapping conditions (e.g., individualized educational programs, accommodations both at home and school to increase structure and consistency, and stimulant medication), although appropriate given our present understanding of learning disabilities, are often inadequate to resolve the primary handicaps. As a result, the child with learning disabilities may not receive the usual "strokes" that go along with school success, and is apt to resort to inappropriate attention-seeking behaviors to get the recognition that otherwise would not be received. Additionally, children with learning disabilities are cognizant of the fact that their performance does not measure up to the standard of the group, resulting in poor self-concept. Inappropriate attention-seeking behaviors and poor self-concept are examples of secondary handicapping conditions that parents and professionals must attempt to prevent or minimize. This chapter presents strategies for managing these secondary behavioral and emotional problems. It is our opinion that implementation of these strategies is most important for ensuring optimal outcome.

MANAGING BEHAVIOR PROBLEMS

Establishing a Behavior Management System

If there are specific behaviors upon which parents and teachers would like to see the child improve, or certain tasks that need to be completed with less supervision, it may be worthwhile to establish a behavior management system. Quite simply, a behavior management system requires that the desired behaviors be specified clearly, that the child's performance on these behaviors be recorded carefully, and that successful performance be rewarded systematically. The key is consistency, both in recording the child's performance and in administering rewards.

Steps are offered for establishing a behavior management system. They are equally appropriate for the home and the classroom. In some cases, parents and teachers may want to work together to create one behavior management system that covers both home and school behaviors. To do this, the teacher might be asked to send home a report each day that tells how many objectives the child accomplished at school. Parents can record on the home behavior management system the child's performance on school objectives. Parents can be responsible for providing a reward at the end of the week if both home and school objectives have been met by the child.

The behavior management system requires a commitment from the parent or teacher who chooses to establish one. A behavior management system should not be attempted by parents or teachers who do not have the motivation or time to carry it through. This situation will only result in the child being taught that parents or teachers do not follow through with their own goals. On the other hand, teachers and parents should remind themselves that it may be easier to work hard to control some undesirable behaviors than to ignore them and have them escalate into more serious problems in the future.

The first step in establishing a behavior management system is to specify the behaviors or tasks upon which the child needs to improve. Objectives for improving the child's behavior and completing tasks should be outlined in writing. To do this, the parent or teacher should list the daily tasks that the child is expected to complete, being as specific as possible. For home behavior management, the list should include the child's assigned chores (e.g., clearing the dinner dishes, emptying waste baskets, feeding pets), as well as other tasks that the child may have difficulty completing independently (e.g., getting ready for school on time, completing homework assignments, taking baths). At school, various regular tasks should be listed (e.g., copying the homework assignment, completing daily assignments in reading, spelling, and arithmetic, participating in social studies discussion). Parents and teachers should be specific regarding their expectations. For example, instead of listing "Get ready for school on time," parents may need to specify "Get dressed, brush teeth, wash hands and face before 7:30 A.M." The list also can include behaviors parents and teachers would like to see the child improve. As much as possible, these should be stated in a positive way. For example, instead of listing "Don't wander around the classroom," the teacher might want to state "Ask permission before leaving your seat." It may be more difficult to specify the behaviors that need improvement than the tasks to be completed, but again teachers and parents should try to be as specific as possible. For example, "Be polite to parents," should not be included as an item. Instead, parents may want to specify "Say please and thank you when appropriate, wait your turn before speaking, and look at your parents when they are speaking to you."

The list of objectives should be discussed with the child. The child should have some input regarding which household chores he or she would prefer and when he or she might prefer doing them. Parents and teachers should discuss with the child the reasons they would like the child to take more responsibility for personal tasks and to improve certain behaviors. The child should not be allowed to dictate the list, but his or her cooperation should be elicited in setting objectives.

In selecting objectives on which to begin the behavior management system, the parent or teacher should choose four or five critical objectives on which to start, together with two or three easy objectives. All of the child's shortcomings cannot be expected to improve at once. Both adult and child will become frustrated if the behavior management system attempts to address too extensive a list of objectives. By initially targeting a few selected critical and easy behaviors, and demonstrating some immediate success with these, parents and teachers will be more likely to maintain motivation for continuing the system, and will generalize the system to deal with additional behaviors in their listings.

For each of the objectives selected, the parent or teacher should set reasonable time limits (if appropriate), criteria for success (if appropriate), and any other limitations or restrictions for successful completion. For example, if the objective is "Start your homework on your own," it may be desirable to set a time limit (e.g., "Before 7:30 P.M."). If the objective is "Complete 25 math problems," a criteria for success can be added (e.g., "with at least 90 percent accuracy"). If the objective is "empty the wastebaskets in all rooms every day," the restriction "without reminders" might be added. Clearly, it is inappropriate to set time limits and criteria for each objective. This should be done only when it helps to clarify the expectations for completion of the objective.

The next step is to set up a checklist where objectives are listed down the side of a sheet of paper, and days of the week are listed across the top of the page. (See Tables 11-1 and 11-2.) If some objectives are to be accomplished only on certain days, x's should be placed in the boxes corresponding to the days on which objectives are not to be completed. The child's successful completion of each objective will be recorded each day, with either a check or sticker in the corresponding box. It is important that the child's performance be recorded consistently every day. Parents and teachers should not wait until the end of the week and try to remember what objectives were achieved each day.

The behavior management system is based on reward for successful completion of objectives. First, parents or teachers need to decide how many of the objectives must be accomplished successfully within a week for the child to earn a specific reward. The behavior management system outlined in Table 11-1 has 26 spaces for recording successful behavior. It is a good idea to start with a fairly easy criteria (e.g., "Eighteen of 26 objectives must be met in order to receive a reward at the end of the week"). The number of objectives selected for criteria will depend on the difficulty of the objectives and on the likelihood that the child will be able to complete them. The number of objectives necessary for reward can be increased as the system continues and the child achieves more success.

The next step is to work with the child in deciding what would be an appropriate reward for successful completion of the prescribed number of objectives. It will be important to provide verbal praise for the completion of each objective every day. However, more tangible reinforcement will be necessary for rewarding the child for success at the end of the week. Parents should not get carried away with promises of expensive toys or activities. They should keep in mind that they may have to provide the reward every week. Some rewards that might be appropriate for the behavior management system at home include:

- [ ] Staying up until midnight on Saturday night to watch a special movie (one that has already been approved)
- [ ] Having a friend spend the night on a weekend
- [ ] Money for roller skating, movie, or bowling

TABLE 11-1

Sample Behavior Management System to Be Used at Home

OBJECTIVES	Mon	Tues	Wed	Thurs	Fri	Sat	Sun
Make bed every morning before 7 A.M. without reminder (10 A.M. on nonschool days).							
Get ready for school (wash face, get dressed, get books and papers together, eat breakfast, brush teeth) before 7:30 A.M. without reminders.						X	X
Take out trash cans on garbage pick-up days before school, with one reminder.	X		X	X		X	X
Keep your hands to yourself when playing with your sister.							
Start homework on your own before 7 P.M. without reminder.						X	X

Criteria for reward: Successful completion of 18 out of 26 objectives.
Reward: Going bowling on Saturday with Dad and a friend.

☐ Purchase of a small toy, perhaps part of a collection the child has started
☐ Going to lunch or on an outing with mom or dad, without siblings

Rewards that might be appropriate for the behavior management system at school include:

☐ A half-hour of "free time" on Friday afternoon
☐ Being selected as the teacher's "special helper" to run errands or help younger students
☐ Being allowed to use special materials for an art project of the child's choice
☐ Being allowed to play with a particular group of educational toys
☐ Participating on a particular class outing

The teacher might also be able to solicit cooperation from parents in providing a reward for appropriate school behavior.

TABLE 11-2
Sample Behavior Management System to Be Used at School

OBJECTIVES	Mon	Tues	Wed	Thurs	Fri	Sat	Sun
Be seated and have materials on your desk by 8:30 A.M.							
Complete daily assignment in arithmetic without supervision, within a 20-minute time limit, with 90% accuracy.							
Ask permission before leaving your seat 90% of the time.							
Participate in social studies discussion by making at least two appropriate comments, without being asked by the teacher.							
Walk quietly in the halls.							

Criteria for reward: Successful completion of 20 out of the 25 objectives.

Reward: One-half hour of "free time" on Friday, to be spent on playground, in the classroom, or in the library.

In selecting a reward, parents and teachers should keep the following in mind:

☐ The reward should be obtainable at the end of the week. Parents should not tell the child, for example, that he or she can have a big reward, such as a bicycle, if he or she succeeds on the objectives for 10 weeks in a row. Similarly, a teacher who promises the child an "A" at the end of the term may not be able to elicit much motivation for the system. Most children cannot delay gratification much longer than a week and will lose interest in the system.

☐ The reward should not be a continuation of privileges the child already has. That is, the child should not be threatened with the removal of existing privileges if he or she does not meet criteria.

☐ Money can be used as a reinforcer if parents desire. However, it is better to earmark the money for a particular purchase so that the child has something to work toward. It is better not to use this with younger children, and probably should be used only if the parent and child cannot think of less mercenary reinforcers.

☐ If possible, reinforcers should be chosen that incorporate values parents and teachers would like to see developed (e.g., family togetherness, sharing with classmates, socializing with friends, physical fitness).

☐ If the child does not meet the criteria, parents and teachers must be consistent in not administering rewards, so they should not select as a reward something they intend for the child to have regardless of his or her behavior (e.g., summer camp, birthday party, class picnic).

It may be necessary with very young children (under 6 years) to provide reinforcement on a daily basis rather than on a weekly basis. If so, the parent or teacher should use the same procedure outlined, but make the reward smaller (e.g., playing a game of the child's choice with mom or dad for a half-hour before going to bed, choosing the story that will be read to the class). The time between reinforcers can gradually be lengthened as the child gets older and begins to have consistent success with the system.

Parents and teachers should make certain the child understands the rules of the system from the outset and understands what the reward will be. If the child thinks something about the system is unfair, the problem should be worked out before starting the system, if possible. The child's success on each objective should be recorded every day. The child can be allowed to put stickers or checks in the boxes on the chart, with supervision.

At the end of the week the parent or teacher should review the child's progress with him or her. If the child does not meet criteria, the parent or teacher should not scold, but should stay calm and say, "We'll try it again next week." (If the system is begun with fairly easy criteria for reinforcement, failure can be avoided in the beginning. Parents and teachers should remember that the objective is to have the child succeed.) The parent or teacher may want to spend some time with the child discussing where he or she experienced the greatest difficulty in meeting the objectives and suggest some ways to help him or her do better next week. If the child has succeeded in reaching the criteria for reinforcement, parents or teachers should provide verbal praise, tell the child how proud they are of his or her accomplishments, and make arrangements for administering the reward as soon as possible. If the child has succeeded in reaching the criteria for reward several weeks in a row, the difficulty for reaching criteria can be increased, either by adding new objectives or by requiring that more of the existing objectives be met each week.

If the child does not reach criteria for reward, no matter how close he or she came, the reward must not be administered. If it is administered, the parent or teacher will be teaching the child to see how little he or she can get away with doing and still get the reward.

In summary, parents or teachers should specify clearly what is expected, the criteria for earning the reward, and what the reward will be. They must be consistent in recording daily performance and in administering the rewards. Plenty of verbal praise should be given along the way. Nagging and criticism should be avoided.

Psychotherapy for Behavior Problems

The two defining characteristics of ADHD are inattention and impulsivity. The child with ADHD often misbehaves because he or she impulsively acts before thinking about the consequences of his or her behavior. Therapists have attempted to modify impulsive behavior through many techniques, including imposed delay, modeling, identification of failures, establishing response cost contingencies, and self-instructional training (Kendall & Finch, 1979). One type of therapy that appears to have good potential for success is cognitive behavior therapy. Using this approach, therapists teach children strategies for thinking before responding. In some cases, modeling, self-instruction, and response-cost contingencies are used as part of the training. Some programs (e.g., the "think aloud" program developed by Camp, Blom, Herbert, & Van Doornenck, 1977) emphasize social behaviors by teaching children to evaluate how their behavior affects others, to develop alternative strategies for addressing conflicts, and to think before acting. As with most therapies, the success of cognitive behavior therapy depends a great deal on the skill of the therapist. Furthermore, the strategies presented during therapy do not always generalize sufficiently to situations outside the therapy session. Despite these common drawbacks of psychotherapy, cognitive behavior therapy appears to be quite appropriate for many children with ADHD, especially those with good verbal skills.

MANAGING SECONDARY EMOTIONAL DISTURBANCE

The most common emotional disturbance observed in children with learning disabilities or ADHD is poor self-concept. After years of academic failure, social failure, and criticism from parents and teachers, this outcome is not at all surprising. Parents and teachers should make efforts to maintain a young child's self-concept before the effects of learning disability and ADHD have a chance to damage it. For the older child whose learning disabilities and ADHD are not diagnosed until after self-concept is damaged, special accommodations will be needed to help the child feel more positive about himself or herself. The following suggestions are appropriate for either maintaining or remediating poor self-concept:

- [ ] The child should be encouraged to participate in structured nonacademic group activities that will allow him or her to compete successfully with peers in areas where he or she is not so far behind. Because so much of the poor self-concept of the child with learning disabilities derives from academic problems at school, it is especially important to identify, if possible, school-related activities in which the child may be expected to succeed (e.g., participation in school athletics, clubs, and offices). All too often the child with learning disabilities is excluded from these activities because of poor grades. These extracurricular activities may be important in drawing the child back into what is inherently a difficult learning process.
- [ ] Parents and teachers should attempt to identify and encourage any special strengths or talents a child might have (e.g., music, art, leadership, creative writing). It is important for the child to be able to achieve success and earn praise for some special skill or talent, especially if academic achievement is not a source of positive reinforcement.
- [ ] Parents should make efforts to identify, encourage, and praise strengths that distinguish the child from siblings, especially if siblings are perceived by the child as more successful.
- [ ] Parents and teachers should make efforts to provide the child with special responsibilities that the child can handle with success. For example, the teacher might regularly ask the child to take messages to the school office, to assist in classroom "chores" (e.g., taking inventory of materials, organizing shelves, taking attendance), to assist younger students, or act as a member of the safety patrol. If possible, the child should be given opportunities that will allow him or her to feel important in the eyes of peers. For example, he or she might be allowed to assist the teacher in directing the class play, teach a lesson on a subject in which he or she has particular expertise, or share a special experience with the class.
- [ ] The child should be praised for good attempts at new activities, regardless of the outcome of these efforts.
- [ ] Parents and teachers should solicit the child's input when planning activities. Whenever possible, the child's suggestions should be incorporated into the plans to make him or her feel that his or her input is valued.

In general, parents and teachers should attempt to make the child feel that he or she is special in a positive sense to overcome all of the negative attention he or she receives as a result of learning disabilities and attention problems. Parents and teachers must become attuned to every opportunity that warrants praise and reinforcement. If strategies for maintaining self-concept are integrated into the educational process as soon as academic difficulties are identified, serious behavioral and emotional problems may be obviated. Sadly, the maintenance of self-concept is sometimes ignored until problems have gotten out of hand. When efforts by teachers and parents are insufficient or delayed, psychotherapy often is necessary. Although poor self-concept is the most common emotional disturbance observed in conjunction with learning disabilities and ADHD, other concomitant disorders can include depression, school phobia, eating disorders, substance abuse, excessive tension, anger, or hostility. Most parents and school personnel are unequipped to deal with these more serious emotional disturbances. In these cases, professional counseling for the child must be sought. The physician may be able to help convince the parent of this need and to assist in selecting an appropriate therapist. Family therapy is often necessary when the child's learning disabilities or ADHD have led to conflict within the family situation.

CONCLUSION

Strategies discussed in Chapters 9 and 10 for dealing with primary handicapping conditions often are inadequate to resolve the problems fully. As a result, the child with learning disabilities often experiences secondary handicapping conditions, including behavior problems and poor self-concept. Strategies for dealing with behavior problems include the establishment of behavior management systems, both at home and school, and, when necessary, psychotherapy. Poor self-concept is addressed through the consistent application of positive reinforcement. If these strategies for handling behavior problems and maintaining self-concept are consistently employed, many of the secondary handicapping conditions can be minimized or avoided altogether.

CHAPTER 12

Life After High School—Promoting Effective Transition for the Adolescent with Learning Disabilities

Nick Elksnin
Linda K. Elksnin

Interest in the unique needs of adolescents with learning disabilities began in the mid to late seventies as professionals realized that, although some manifestations of learning disabilities could be lessened through remedial and compensatory strategies, learning disabilities could not be "cured." Only recently have parents and professionals acknowledged the need to prepare young persons with learning disabilities to make the successful transition from high school to postsecondary training and/or employment. Our ultimate goal for individuals with learning disabilities following high school is 100 percent integration in employment settings, nonbaccalaureate programs, or baccalaureate programs. However, only approximately 60 percent of students with learning disabilities graduate from high school, with about half of this number earning a high school diploma (as opposed to successfully meeting Individualized Education Program objectives, but failing to meet graduation requirements). Results of the National Transition Study (Wagner, 1989) which followed approximately 8,000 youths ages 13 to 23 with handicaps, indicated only 16 percent of students with learning disabilities entered postsecondary training programs, with 1.6

percent enrolled in four-year colleges and universities, 4.9 percent in two-year colleges, and 1.1 percent in vocational schools. Sitlington and Frank (1990) surveyed individuals with learning disabilities a year following graduation and reported that only 54 percent made a successful transition to adult life. Individuals making successful transitions were employed or engaged in postsecondary training activities, were at least partially self-supporting, and involved in more than one leisure activity. Employment outcome data are no more encouraging. Results of follow-up studies indicate that individuals with learning disabilities tend to be underemployed and unemployed more frequently than their nondisabled peers.

SECONDARY PROGRAM MODELS

For students with learning disabilities to make smooth transitions to employment or postsecondary training, they must be placed in secondary learning disabilities programs that are compatible with transition goals. In the following sections we review prevalent secondary programs, including *remediation, tutorial, compensatory, strategies intervention,* and *work-study* models. The compatibility of each model with effective transition is considered.

The Basic Skills Remediation Model is an extension of the predominant elementary model. Basic skills in reading, mathematics, and written expression continue to be taught to adolescents with learning disabilities who failed to master these skills as elementary students. Although we do not discount the importance of being able to read and perform rudimentary mathematics calculations, we would argue that teaching academics for academics sake at the secondary level does little to promote use of these skills in real life situations. Secondary students who are significantly deficient in basic math and reading skills are unlikely to respond dramatically to basic skills instruction, leaving them ill-equipped to read or solve rudimentary mathematics problems or to pursue postsecondary training or employment following high school.

In the *Tutorial Model,* the learning disability specialist tutors the student in regular education classes. For example, the student (or the student's regular education teacher) may request that the learning disability specialist help the student prepare for a unit test in U.S. history, learn a list of vocabulary words for the English quiz, or help the student learn to solve simple algebraic equations. Many leaders in the field of learning disabilities have referred to the tutorial model as a band-aid approach which results in students becoming dependent rather than independent learners. The student may pass a test, but continues to lack skills required to be successful on future exams. The tutorial model does little to facilitate successful transition to postsecondary training or employment. Although tutorial services may supplement learning disability services for students requiring them, we question the use of a highly trained learning disability specialist for this purpose. Peer tutoring or tutoring provided by school volunteers are reasonable alternatives, permitting the specialist to assist the student to become an independent learner.

The previous two models focus on improving the learner's skills or knowledge. *The Compensatory Model* relies on changing the student's instructional environment. Modifications and accommodations are made with regard to how content is presented and evaluated. Presentation modifications might include delivering content through films and demonstration in addition to lecture and reading assignments. Evaluation modifications include permitting the student with learning disabilities to demonstrate competence through demonstration or successful completion of an oral examination. This model may promote successful transition if students become aware of their learning characteristics and are able to request appropriate environmental modifications in postsecondary settings.

Don Deshler, Jean Schumaker, and their colleagues at the University of Kansas Institute for Research in Learning Disabilities developed an alternative model. The Strategies Intervention Model (SIM) is designed to enable students with learning disabilities to become more efficient and effective learners. The *Learning Strategies Curriculum* of SIM enables secondary level students to learn *how* to learn rather than *what* to learn. Students are taught strategies that are applied across academic and vocational content areas. Strategies that enable students to decode multisyllabic words, find the main idea of a passage, take notes, write themes, and take tests more efficiently enable students to become independent learners. SIM promotes effective transition to postsecondary training or employment by teaching students with learning disabilities strategies that generalize across settings, foster student independence,and help students become their own advocates.

The Work Study Model advocates direct teaching of job-related academic skills. For example, for the student with learning disabilities enrolled in a carpentry program, measuring actual objects to the sixteenth of an inch may be more appropriate than having the student measure lines on a ditto sheet to the nearest quarter inch. This model requires collaboration between the learning disability specialist and the vocational educator. The model can facilitate successful transition to the world of work or postsecondary vocational training programs.

LEGISLATION AFFECTING TRANSITION EFFORTS

Public Law 94-142, The Education for All Handicapped Children Act of 1975, requires that vocational education be made available to school-age students with handicaps. The act defines vocational education as:

> organized educational programs which are directly related to the preparation of individuals for paid or unpaid employment, or for the additional preparation for a career requiring other than a baccalaureate or advanced degree (Public Law 94-142, 34 C.F.R. 121 [A] [11]).

Two other pieces of legislation also are relevant to secondary and postsecondary training designed to enable students with learning disabilities to be successful adults: Section 504 of the Rehabilitation Act and the Carl D. Perkins Vocational Education Act.

Enacted in 1973, Section 504 often is referred to as the civil rights law for persons with handicaps. The act prohibits an institution that receives federal funds from discriminating against otherwise qualified individuals with disabilities. Institutions include schools, colleges, universities, and places of employment. The courts have interpreted "otherwise qualified" to mean that the individual must be able to meet all essential requirements for the job or postsecondary training program in spite of the handicap. Employers and educators, however, must make "reasonable accommodation" to allow the person with the handicap to meet the requirements. Section 504 essentially mandates equal educational opportunities for individuals with learning disabilities in colleges and universities because most institutions receive federal assistance in the form of financial aid to students. This legislation not only has implications for recruitment and admission of qualified students with learning disabilities to postsecondary institutions, but also impacts upon program and activity accessibility. There is no official federal interpretation of "reasonable accommodations," but states, colleges, and universities have interpreted this requirement in ways which suggest that reasonable modifications of academic requirements include: (a) course substitutions, (b) modifying or waiving foreign language requirements, (c) additional time to complete degree programs, and (d) permitting part-time rather than full-time study.

The Carl D. Perkins Vocational Education Act, legislated in 1984, enables students who are handicapped and disadvantaged to access the full range of vocational programs available to individuals who are not handicapped. Students with learning disabilities who are enrolled in vocational programs are entitled under this Act to have their interests, abilities, and special needs assessed; instruction, equipment, and curricula modified to meet their special needs; counseling services needed to enable them to make a smooth transition from school to post-school employment and career opportunities. In addition, students must receive appropriate guidance, counseling, and career development activities during their secondary careers. In 1990, the Perkins Act was amended and renamed the Carl D. Perkins Vocational and Applied Technology Act. This legislation takes a broader view of vocational education and regards it as a means of acquiring higher level thinking and academic skills in addition to learning occupational skills. The amendments also differ from the original legislation in that a clear distinction is made between secondary and postsecondary levels of vocational education, with separate funding mechanisms for each level.

In our discussion of transition of adolescents with learning disabilities which follows, we consider transition needs of those students who obtain employment immediately following high school and of those students who desire postsecondary training.

MAKING THE TRANSITION FROM HIGH SCHOOL TO EMPLOYMENT

The goal for some students with learning disabilities is to get and keep a job immediately following high school. For this goal to be achieved, students must have access to effective vocational programs. Sitlington (1986) identified three vocational education program models which typically are used to serve students with learning disabilities. When students enter vocational programs designed for regular education students, professionals either have attempted to *change the system, assist the learner to fit the system,* or *ignore the system.* The first model is dependent upon the special education teacher providing consultation to the vocational educator regarding the types of appropriate instructional modifications. Several approaches have been used to enable the student with learning disabilities to fit into the existing vocational program more effectively. The student may receive in-class assistance from support personnel such as the learning disabilities specialist. The specialist may provide instruction in the resource room which supplements the vocational teachers' instruction in much the same way the student is tutored in academic subject areas. The learner also may receive instruction in generalizable skills designed to complement the vocational program. Generalizable skills are academic and interpersonal skills which appear to generalize across vocational programs. A third model bypasses the system by creating a separate vocational program for students with learning disabilities. This third option has become less popular because of the desire to educate students with learning disabilities in the least restrictive environment (i.e., with their nonhandicapped peers). However, for some students with severe learning disabilities an intensive self-contained vocational training program that utilizes job coaches may be appropriate.

ROLES OF PROFESSIONALS AND FAMILIES

In this chapter we advocate collaboration among professionals, parents, and students to promote effective transition from high school to employment (Elksnin & Elksnin, 1990). Individuals representing different disciplines and/or agencies are instrumental in assuring that students with learning disabilities make a smooth postsecondary transition (Feichtner, 1989; Sitlington, 1986).

Vocational Educators

Vocational educators provide specific vocational training and assist in locating vocational training sites for those individuals who desire postsecondary training. Vocational educators also may collect vocational assessment data and develop vocational Individualized Education Plan (IEP) and Individualized Transition Plan (ITP) objectives.

Special Educators

Special educators collect and analyze assessment data, provide consultation regarding program modification, provide supplementary instruction as needed, and educate the community regarding the capabilities of individuals with learning disabilities, and coordinate transition planning.

Vocational Rehabilitation Counselors

Until 1981, individuals with learning disabilities were excluded from vocational rehabilitation eligibility because learning disability was not regarded as a mental or physical disability. Vocational Rehabilitation considers "individuals who have a disorder in one or more of the psychological processes involved in understanding, perceiving, or expressing language or concepts (spoken or written)" as learning

disabled (P. L. 94-142, 34 C. F. R. 300.5 [b] [9]). To qualify for services, the individual with learning disabilities must meet these criteria:
  a. Their psychological processing disorder is diagnosed by a licensed physician an/or a licensed or certified psychologist who is skilled in the diagnosis and treatment of such disorders; and
  b. Their disorder results in a substantial handicap to employment; and
  c. There is a reasonable expectation that vocational rehabilitation services may benefit the individual in terms of employability. (Office of Information and Resources for the Handicapped, 1980 [p. 4])

Vocational rehabilitation counselors can secure funding for job-related services such as on-site training, provide vocational evaluation information, facilitate job placement and provide support services, and educate the community to promote integration of persons with learning disabilities in community job settings. The Vocational Rehabilitation Act Amendments of 1984 require that counselors serve secondary-level students who are attempting to make the transition from school to work. Vocational Rehabilitation services include vocational training, academic support services, medical treatment, educational and medical evaluations, and other support services such as transportation, books, tools, and so forth.

Employers

Employers assist in transition by making job training sites and employment available. Information about job requirements and employer needs is useful when developing and enhancing learning disability and vocational programs. Employers' prescriptions of secondary and postsecondary support services are useful when developing these services or evaluating existing services.

Parents

Parents contribute to the transition process by helping their adolescent child with learning disabilities develop realistic career goals and helping develop Individualized Education Plan and Individualized Transition Plan goals. It is essential that parents be supportive as the adolescent with learning disabilities explores career and employment options. Parents can foster independence by providing structure and encouragement and by allowing the adolescent with learning disabilities to assume responsibility for home and school tasks.

Students

The adolescent with learning disabilities must assume a high level of responsibility for developing and reaching transition goals. Secondary learning disability and vocational programs that promote independence and responsibility will assist the student in assuming the role of self-advocate. One approach that can be used to encourage students to become more involved in their Individualized Education Plans and Individualized Transition Plans is the *Education Planning Strategy* developed by the University of Kansas (Van Reusen, Bos, Schumaker, & Deshler, 1987). *I PLAN* is a motivational strategy students can use as they prepare for or participate in IEP and ITP meetings. *I PLAN* includes these five steps: *I*nventory strengths, weaknesses, goals, and learning choices, *P*rovide inventory information to others at the meeting, *L*isten and respond to others, *A*sk questions during the meeting, and *N*ame your goals.

MAKING THE TRANSITION TO COLLEGE

During the past decade, the number of students with learning disabilities in college has increased tenfold. Many of these students, however, never complete their college degree programs. It is important that high school learning disability programs enable students with learning disabilities to acquire the skills they will require in college settings: course content, study skills, self-reliance, self-knowledge, and self-advocacy. Secondary teachers and parents must create situations that foster student independence. College transition is a three-stage process: from secondary school to college, from college entrance to college graduation, and from college graduation to employment.

From Secondary School To College

During this stage, students and their parents need information about college options. Information can be obtained through printed materials, workshops, and forums. Students with learning disabilities need a clear understanding of the basic differences between high school and college. Stan Shaw and his colleagues at the University of Connecticut identified several basic differences, including the amount of time in class (e.g., 6 hours per day for 180 days for high school versus 12 hours per week for 28 weeks for college), study time (more required in college), testing practices (e.g., tests are administered less frequently in college), teacher expectations (e.g., college faculty demand a higher level of independence), and structure (e.g., the high degree of externally imposed structure in high school versus the self-determined structure of college).

Siperstein (1988) also recommends that an Individualized College Plan (ICP) be developed that will enable students to be aware of their strengths and weaknesses, the types of instructional accommodations they may require, the availability of educational and financial resources, and so on. The ICP can be used to develop a plan that will enable students to overcome personal, environmental, and social obstacles to success in college.

When selecting a college for the student with learning disabilities, Strichart and Mangrum (1985) suggest that students and parents closely examine the institution's admission policy. Some colleges will consider results from individual intelligence tests to determine if a student has the aptitude for college. Others will consider subtest scores from alternative administrations (e.g., taped, untimed) of the Scholastic Aptitude Test to evaluate an applicant with learning disabilities. The admissions process may allow for letters of support from content area teachers and on-campus interviews. In addition, the availability of these services should be determined: diagnostic and prescriptive planning, special advisement, remediation of basic skills, tutoring, special courses to acquire critical skills (e.g., study, communication, composition), auxiliary aids and services such as taped textbooks, and counseling services.

The goal of college selection should be to match the student to the institution. A formal procedure which facilitates this process is the *McGuire-Shaw Postsecondary Guide for Learning* that considers the characteristics of students, the institution, and available learning disabilities support programs. Appendix B includes a list of college learning disabilities guides.

From College Entrance To College Graduation

Success in college for the student with learning disabilities may require a combination of changing the student to match the institution and changing the institution to match the student.

Changing the Student

The college student with learning disabilities may require programs that remediate basic skills and provide academic tutoring. Students may need instruction in study skills and access to learning aids such as taped textbooks and notetakers. The academic and social adjustment of the student may be assisted through individual and group counseling services. Students with learning disabilities may need assistance in selecting courses, beyond the help normally provided by a college advisor. An appropriate match between student and course can be achieved by considering the student's learning characteristics with the course materials, content presentation, methods of evaluation, and classroom standards (Patton & Polloway, 1987). Finally, students need to learn self-advocacy techniques including sitting in front, asking to tape a lecture, planning assignments in advance, explaining one's learning difficulties to the instructor, asking the instructor for assistance, and going to all classes and being on time.

Changing the Environment

Often a primary role of the college learning disabilities specialist is to liaison with faculty as modifications such as extended time for tests and assignment completion, provision of lecture notes, use of audiovisual equipment, and adjustment of grading standards often initially meet with resistance. College faculty need to become more sensitive to the needs of students with learning disabilities. Figure 12-1 provides a list of instructional accommodations for college students with learning disabilities that can be provided by college faculty.

Another important function of college learning disabilities services is to identify institutional resources that may be beneficial to students with learning disabilities. These resources may include library services such as books on tape, audiovisual aids, and other special equipment; student services such as personal counseling, career/life planning, health services; and learning labs such as writing centers, reading labs, study skills centers, and computer-assisted instruction (see Figure 12-2).

In addition to instructional modifications and accessibility to resources, institutional policy changes may lead to more adaptive environments for the student with learning disabilities. Although not widespread, these policy changes may include modification of admissions requirements, specially designed courses, semester load reductions, and foreign language waivers or substitutions.

Students preparing to make the transition from college to employment will require ongoing career counseling. As graduation draws nearer, the college student with learning disabilities will need to learn job search and job maintenance strategies.

FIGURE 12-1.
Instructional Accommodations For College Students With Learning Disabilities

TEACHING STRATEGIES

Provide students with advance organizers such as outlines, schedule of due dates for projects, reading assignments, and exams.

Give students an outline prior to lecture.

Use handouts to list important terms, formulas, key points, and so on.

Write and define new terms on the board.

Provide oral summary statement of key points.

Read material written on board or on overhead transparencies.

Permit the student to use a notetaker.

Allow the student to photocopy another student's notes.

Permit the student to tape record the lecture.

Encourage class discussion.

Provide positive and negative examples.

ASSISTING STUDENTS IN THEIR READING AND WRITTEN WORK

Provide students with chapter outlines or study guides.

Permit students to use a dictionary, computer spell check, or proofreader.

Allow students to use readers, scribes, word processors, tape recorders, and typewriters.

Permit students to use a calculator in math or science classes.

Allow students additional time to complete written assignments.

EVALUATION STRATEGIES

Allow students to complete paper and project drafts for critique; permit rewriting.

Give students additional time to complete examinations.

Allow students time to study before administering an examination or quiz.

Be sure examination questions are well-spaced on the page.

Avoid requiring student to transfer responses to an answer sheet.

Allow students to take examination as an oral essay, to tape answers, or to use a transcriber for essay exams.

Allow poor grammar on exams if grammar is not the primary focus.

Permit student to take exam with a proctor in a quiet room without distractions.

Administer short exams frequently rather than one or two lengthy exams.

Divide exam and assess student over multiple sessions.

Provide cues to help students recall information. Consider retesting students.

Be willing to consider a variety of test designs (e.g., essay, multiple choice, matching, true-false).

Consider the use of alternatives to test when evaluating student performance (e.g., demonstrations, taped interviews, slide-tape presentations, photographic essays, and so on).

Allow extra credit assignments.

Be willing to schedule individual conferences during the semester to discuss the student's progress.

FIGURE 12-2.
Institutional Resources For College Students With Learning Disabilities

PERSONNEL
Special Education Faculty
LD Administrator/Coordinator
LD Specialists
Notetakers
Peer Tutors
Readers
Scribes
SERVICES
Academic Counseling
Access to computers, tapes, taping, videos, etc.
Career Counseling
Diagnostic Services
Personal Counseling
Self-Help Groups
Tutoring
SPECIAL COURSES
Compensatory/Learning Strategies Instruction
Developmental/Remedial Courses
Social/Interpersonal Skills Training
Study Skills Courses
FACULTY AND STAFF TRAINING
Faculty Awareness Activities
Staff Training

CONCLUSION

Individuals involved in transition planning for adolescents with learning disabilities should be aware of the feelings and needs of students and their parents. Parents may recognize the need to allow their child with learning disabilities to become less dependent upon them, but may have difficulty facilitating independence. The failures and frustrations encountered during the high school years may cause parents to feel apprehensive about their child becoming employed or entering a postsecondary training program. Parents also may anticipate a sense of loss of the familiar educational support system available throughout the elementary and secondary years. For the student with learning disabilities, concerns may relate to lack of postsecondary knowledge and self-advocacy skills and the need to become fully accepting of their learning disability. The learning disability specialist can promote transition for parents and students through these activities (Ness, 1989):

- [ ] Obtaining more information about postsecondary options.
- [ ] Inservicing regular education teachers and guidance teachers to enable them to contribute to the transition process.
- [ ] Assisting the student to understand learning disabilities, to identify personal strengths and weaknesses, and to self-advocate based upon this knowledge.
- [ ] Assist parents in understanding their child's learning disabilities so they can, in turn, encourage the child's self-awareness.
- [ ] Providing support groups and workshops for parents which might feature speakers from advocacy organizations such as the Learning Disability Association of America and the Department of Vocational Rehabilitation Services.
- [ ] Include transition objectives in the student's IEP and begin the transition process by at least the 9th grade through offering the appropriate coursework and career development activities.

CHAPTER 13

The Summary Conference

Frank R. Brown, III
Elizabeth H. Aylward

The goal of the interdisciplinary team process, as described in the preceding chapters, is to develop a consensus opinion regarding diagnoses and to formulate a comprehensive treatment plan. An equally essential element of the diagnostic and prescriptive process is to convey findings and recommendations of the interdisciplinary team to the parents (and, when appropriate, to the child) through a summary conference. The individual assigned this responsibility (usually the case manager) has a very difficult and important responsibility; this is the subject of the final chapter.

In theory, and in the best of circumstances, any professional participating in the interdisciplinary team process should be capable of functioning as case manager and could be assigned the responsibility of explaining the diagnoses and therapeutic recommendations to the parents and child. It is imperative, however, that the case manager understand, at least to a reasonably complete degree, all the factors involved in formulating the interdisciplinary diagnoses and therapeutic recommendations. It is not sufficient for the case manager to understand only his or her own discipline's perspective, as the result would reflect this limited perspective and bias. The person conducting the summary conference should have a good breadth of understanding of the child with learning disabilities and his or her family, and should be able to articulate the team's findings and recommendations to the family in a comprehensive, unbiased, and sensitive way. In particularly difficult cases, it may be beneficial to have several team members present at the summary conference to support the case manager's presentation.

The case manager may want to begin the conference by asking the parents to reiterate the concerns and goals they had at the time the evaluation was initiated. Concerns of the individual who initiated the referral (if not the parents) also should be discussed. With these concerns and goals in mind, the case manager can conduct a conference that will produce appropriate closure on the parent's agenda and, when necessary, expand this agenda to reflect additional diagnostic concerns and therapeutic recommendations from the team's perspective.

PRESENTATION OF THE DIAGNOSES

Throughout this book we have attempted to clearly distinguish between primary (neurologically based) and secondary (derivative of primary) handicapping conditions. It is important that the case manager share this distinction with the parents. By making this distinction, the case manager provides the parents and child with a logical and effective framework for the discussion of diagnoses and therapeutic recommendations.

Diagnoses of Primary Handicapping Conditions

In presenting the team's diagnostic data, the case manager will need to define some terms for the parents, especially the term *learning disability*. Throughout this book, *learning disability* has been defined as a discrepancy between cognitive ability and academic achievement, assuming that other conditions have been ruled out (see Chapter 1). It is important that parents understand the difference between intelligence and academic achievement, because many will presume that these concepts are one and the same. The difference between intelligence and academic achievement sometimes can be explained by describing the types of tasks presented on tests of intelligence (which are presumed to reflect underlying cognitive ability) and tests of academic achievement (which reflect the level of mastery of academic skills).

Following definition of terms, the case manager should review the data from the individual evaluations and highlight those findings that support or refute the diagnosis of a specific learning disability. The case manager can begin by describing any delays in early development that often correlate with subsequent learning disabilities (see Chapter 2). This explanation will help the parents understand the long-standing developmental basis of their child's primary handicapping conditions.

Next, the case manager will present data regarding potential for academic achievement, as defined by the results of the psychologist's formal cognitive assessment. Overall cognitive assessment should be discussed, as well as any significant strengths and weaknesses within the cognitive profile (see Chapter 4).

When discussing the child's academic achievement, it is important to present both the results of the formal achievement tests and the classroom teachers' present and past perspectives on the child's rate of progress (see Chapter 5). Strengths and weaknesses within the academic achievement profile also should be discussed with the parents.

After the case manager has explained the defining characteristics of learning disabilities and has outlined any significant discrepancies between cognitive ability and academic achievement, the diagnostic conclusion regarding the presence or absence of learning disabilities should be quite clear to the parents. Definition of relevant individual learning disabilities (dyslexia, dyscalculia, dysgraphia) will further clarify the diagnosis (see Chapter 1). The case manager should help the parents understand how the learning disabilities will interfere with school performance and how the disabilities may prevent the child from learning through traditional approaches.

Following discussion of learning disabilities, the case manager should introduce any other primary handicapping conditions diagnosed by the team (e.g., attention-deficit hyperactivity disorder [ADHD], language disabilities, fine and gross motor dyscoordination). As with the discussion of learning disabilities, the case manager will need to clearly define the terms associated with each individual diagnosis. Then, data to support or refute each diagnosis should be presented. This data will include test results as well as information obtained through the teacher interview, parent interview, classroom observation, and observation of the child during testing. The case manager should explain how these associated primary conditions will interfere with school performance. For example, parents should be able to easily understand that ADHD may result in inconsistent application to task, fluctuating academic performance, and failure to follow directions.

Diagnoses of Secondary Handicapping Conditions

The case manager should next focus discussion on any secondary handicapping conditions that have been diagnosed or are suspected (e.g., poor self-esteem, behavioral problems). Their definitions, diagnostic features, and implications should be discussed. Data relevant to these conditions may include test results, but more typically will involve information obtained through interviews and observation.

At this point, it will be helpful for the case manager to review the relevant diagnoses and their definitions, and to discuss the relationships among the diagnosed conditions. Parents should understand that the primary handicapping conditions are neurologically based, whereas secondary handicapping conditions probably have occurred as a result of the primary disabilities.

It is especially important that the case manager clarify the distinction between primary and secondary handicapping conditions when discussing ADHD and attention-seeking behavior (see Chapter 10). It should be emphasized that ADHD represents a primary disability frequently associated with learning disabilities, which is to a large extent out of the child's control. This is contrasted with attention-seeking behaviors, which are frequently a secondary condition representing the child's underlying frustration in dealing with the primary handicapping conditions. These attention-seeking behaviors can, with assistance, be brought under the child's willful control. Although these conditions often overlap and may be difficult to disentangle, it is important that the parents understand the distinction between them before therapeutic recommendations are presented.

PRESENTATION OF THERAPEUTIC RECOMMENDATIONS

Following explanation of the diagnoses, the parents' first question probably will be "What do we do about these problems?" The case manager should attempt to respond to this question by systematically reviewing the types of treatment and accommodations appropriate for each specific diagnosis. In discussing these recommendations, the case manager will find it helpful to again use a format based on the distinction between primary and secondary handicapping conditions.

Therapeutic Recommendations for Primary Handicapping Conditions

The case manager should present the team's therapeutic recommendations by first discussing the relatively straightforward procedures used to address the learning disabilities. The issue of special education services should be presented by explaining to parents that their child's learning disabilities prevent him or her from being taught effectively using traditional approaches. Parents should be provided with information regarding the types of special education services that might be available through the school and introduced to the procedures for obtaining these services. Following this general introduction, the case manager should discuss with the parents some of the specialized terminology they will encounter when they meet with the Individual Educational Plan (IEP) development team at their child's school. Some of this terminology will be used in discussing the amount of time the child spends in special programming (e.g., resource classroom, levels of special education service). Other terms will be used in discussing special education methods to which the child will be exposed (e.g., Direct Instruction, Strategies Intervention Model). It is important that parents be familiar with these terms, as this type of "jargon" often is used by school personnel during the IEP development conference without adequate explanation. If the interdisciplinary team wishes to recommend other educational treatment (e.g., tutoring, vocational education) or alternative school placements, these options should also be presented.

Next, the case manager should discuss any special accommodations that the child's teachers (regular or special education) will need to make to circumvent additional primary handicapping conditions often associated with learning disabilities. For example, if the child's handwriting is slow and inefficient, the parents need to understand what types of accommodations the child's teachers should be making (see Chapter 9). Similarly, if the child has ADHD the parents should expect special classroom accommodations to be implemented (see Chapter 10).

The case manager also should discuss the parents' role in the management of primary handicapping conditions, especially ADHD. Specific suggestions for home management of the child (see Chapter 10) should be reviewed with the parents. Strategies for helping the child with homework, organizational difficulties, or other problems associated with the primary handicapping conditions also should be presented.

If the interdisciplinary team (with input from the child's physician) has determined that a trial of medication for ADHD is warranted, the case manager will want to convey this recommendation to the parents. The case manager, depending on his or her familiarity with the medication, may want to provide a full discussion of this topic or may instead want to recommend that the parents speak with the child's physician. In any case, it should always be made clear that the final decision regarding use of medication is to be made by the parents and the child's physician.

Therapeutic Recommendations for Secondary Handicapping Conditions

Therapeutic recommendations for the prevention or treatment of secondary handicapping conditions should be presented following discussion of the primary handicapping conditions. This area of discussion is most important because these secondary handicapping conditions, unlike the primary conditions, almost always can be prevented or eliminated, if parents and teachers deal with the child appropriately.

During the evaluation, the interdisciplinary team will have identified inappropriate attention-seeking behaviors that are a cause for concern among parents or teachers. The case manager should explain to the parents how they can help the child control these behaviors through a behavior management system (see Chapter 11). It may be necessary in some cases for the parents and school to coordinate their efforts in establishing a single behavior management system that covers inappropriate behaviors both at home and school. Strategies for establishing such a system should be discussed with the parents.

Finally, and perhaps most importantly, the case manager should discuss strategies for maintaining or improving the child's self-concept. This area is of vital importance because, when all is said and done, the child's image of himself or herself and his or her ability to relate to others are probably the greatest determinants of overall success.

Parents need to understand their role in building the child's self-concept. They should be encouraged to implement some of the specific strategies discussed in Chapter 11 (e.g., identifying and encouraging special strengths or talents, encouraging participation in structured nonacademic group activities). More importantly, they can accept the fact that the basis of many of the child's difficulties is neurological and, therefore, out of the child's control. When parents stop holding the child accountable for learning difficulties, attention problems, and poor impulse control, and focus on providing the extra structure and support needed, the child's self-concept will improve.

Parents also need to understand the school's responsibility for building the child's self-concept. They may need to work as the child's advocate to make certain that each year teachers are making the special accommodations necessary to allow the child maximum success.

ANSWERING PARENTS' QUESTIONS

Through a systematic approach of defining terms, presenting data to support or refute diagnoses, explaining how each handicapping condition will interfere with performance, and presenting therapeutic recommendations to treat or accommodate each condition, the case manager should be able to convey to the parents a fairly comprehensive understanding of their child's situation. Regardless of the case manager's skills at conveying this information, parents will no doubt have many unanswered questions. The most common of these involve the etiology and prognosis of the disorders.

Discussion of Etiology of Disorders

As discussed in Chapter 1, we view learning disabilities and associated primary handicapping conditions as neurologically based. With an understanding of the neurological basis of learning disabilities, parents are sometimes better able to recognize that the child is not at fault and cannot be held responsible for his or her difficulties. Because neurological damage in children with learning disabilities is quite subtle and diffuse, the cause of this damage cannot, in most cases, be determined for certain. Parents should be discouraged from dwelling on "what went wrong," as determination of the precise etiology of the disorders usually is not possible nor requisite in their treatment.

Discussion of Prognosis of Disorders

Parents almost always want to know "Will my child get better?" The answer to this question almost always can be answered affirmatively, because the child will continue to develop and make academic progress. (The exception to this rule would be the child whose self-concept and attitude toward school have been damaged beyond recovery.)

However, if the question is phrased "Will my child be normal?" the answer cannot be as reassuring. The neurological damage or dysfunction believed to underlie learning disabilities and concomitant conditions will not disappear. It is known, however, that certain areas of the brain can compensate for damage that has occurred in other areas. In addition, children with learning disabilities (especially those who are bright) will learn strategies to compensate for areas of weakness. Unfortunately, it is not possible to determine the extent to which compensation will occur and it is, therefore, not possible to determine to what extent functions eventually will appear normal. Parents often are told that their children will "outgrow" the primary handicapping conditions, especially ADHD, around the time of puberty. The case manager should caution parents that this expectation is usually unrealistic.

Despite the fact that the neurological damage or dysfunction underlying primary handicapping conditions cannot be changed, parents should not be left with the idea that remedial efforts are worthless. Special education teachers can help children with learning disabilities develop strategies for compensating or working around their learning handicaps. Counselors can sometimes help children with ADHD apply strategies for controlling their impulsivity. Occupational or physical therapists may be able to help the child find easier methods for accomplishing difficult motor tasks. Despite "specialists'" claims to the contrary and parents' desire for a "normal" child, the current level of understanding of learning disabilities and concomitant conditions does not permit a "cure," and parents should not expect special education teachers or therapists to be able to totally remediate the disorders.

Although special education teachers and therapists cannot be expected to completely remediate learning disabilities and concomitant conditions, they do play an important role in determining how the child learns to accept and handle his or her disabilities. As we have emphasized several times, prevention or remediation of secondary handicapping conditions in children with learning disabilities, especially inappropriate attention-seeking behaviors and poor self-concept, are vital in determining eventual outcome. Placement in special education classes where the child is presented with materials appropriate to his or her achievement level will allow the child to experience success he or she would be unable to achieve in a regular classroom. Accommodations for poor handwriting, poor organizational skills, or attention problems will allow the child the opportunity to demonstrate what he or she is capable of doing, preventing unnecessary frustration. By implementing these strategies, as well as special techniques for handling secondary handicapping conditions, parents and teachers will be able to ensure the best possible outcome for the child with learning disabilities.

PLANNING FOR FOLLOW-UP

Parents should leave the summary conference with the understanding that the interdisciplinary team will monitor implementation of the therapeutic suggestions, conduct regular evaluations of the child's progress, and revise the treatment plan as necessary. If possible, the case manager should outline for the parents any specific tasks they are expected to accomplish (e.g., meeting with the IEP development team, contacting tutors, consulting with the child's pediatrician regarding trial medication for ADHD, implementing behavior management strategies). The case manager should, of course, provide as much assistance as necessary to ensure that the parents will be able to accomplish these tasks. In addition, the case manager should outline the tasks to be completed or monitored by the interdisciplinary team (e.g., preparing the IEP, helping the teacher develop a behavior management system, coordinating a medication trial with the school nurse).

The case manager should outline for the parents what types of future evaluations should be conducted (e.g., academic achievement testing only, complete psychoeducational reevaluation, additional testing by allied professionals) and when. Parents should know that the school automatically will conduct evaluations on a regular basis as long as the child receives special education. If the interdisciplinary team feels additional testing is necessary (to be conducted either through the school or privately), arrangements should be made to ensure that this occurs.

Regardless of the case manager's ability to clearly present definitions, data, diagnoses, and recommendations, parents are bound to have further questions and concerns after they leave the conference. Problems often arise as parents, teachers, and therapists experiment with various strategies for dealing with the child's disorders. The case manager should make certain that the parents feel free to contact him or her for further discussion, advice, or assistance.

CONCLUSION

This chapter has addressed the case manager's important role in conveying the results and recommendations of the interdisciplinary team process. It is suggested that the case manager present diagnoses and therapeutic recommendations using a format that clearly distinguishes between primary and secondary handicapping conditions. To help parents fully understand their child's disorders, the case manager must clearly define diagnostic terms, present data obtained through the evaluations that are relevant to each diagnosis, integrate the data to explain how each diagnosis was formulated, and describe how the disorders will interfere with normal functioning. Therapeutic recommendations relevant to each specific diagnosis (of both primary and secondary handicapping conditions) are then presented. Common questions regarding the etiology and prognosis of learning disabilities and concomitant conditions are discussed, with special emphasis given to the importance of preventing secondary handicapping conditions. The case manager should make certain that parents leave the summary conference with the assurance that the interdisciplinary team will monitor implementation of the therapeutic recommendations, regularly evaluate the child's progress, and revise the treatment plan as necessary. It is hoped that these procedures will make the parent feel that the interdisciplinary team has worked and will continue to work as the child's advocate in obtaining the support and understanding he or she needs for optimal outcome.

Glossary, Appendices, References, and Reference List of Tests

GLOSSARY

Attention-Deficit Hyperactivity Disorder Developmentally inappropriate lack of attention with associated poor impulse control and excessive motor activity.

Criterion-Referenced Test A test designed to determine whether the child has mastered specific skills. Unlike scores from norm-referenced tests, scores from criterion-referenced tests do not reflect comparison of the student with peers.

Dyscalculia Poor achievement in arithmetic compared with overall cognitive ability.

Dyseidetic (Dyslexic) A proposed subtype of reading disability, whereby the child has difficulty remembering the visual configurations of letters and words. Dyseidetic dyslexics spell and read words by their sounds and consequently read very slowly, as they must sound out each word as they go.

Dysgraphia Poor achievement in written language compared with overall cognitive ability.

Dyslexia Difficulty with reading, manifesting as a significant discrepancy between reading achievement and expectations based on cognitive potential.

Dysphonetic (Dyslexic) A proposed subtype of reading disability, whereby the child has difficulty relating symbols to sounds, and consequently, difficulty mastering phonetic word analysis. Dysphonetic dyslexics are dependent on their sight word (visually memorized) vocabulary and make bizarre spelling errors unrelated to the sound of the word.

Dyspraxia Poor praxis or motor planning.

Educational Quotient (EQ) A score that reflects the expected level of academic achievement. The EQ is based on a measure of intellectual functioning and takes into account the statistical phenomenon known as regression toward the mean.

Environmental Accommodations Changes made in the home and school environment to minimize or eliminate the effects of primary handicapping conditions, especially attention deficit disorder.

Error of Measurement An individual's "true score" on a given test is the average of the scores he or she would obtain if the test were given an infinite number of times without any effects from retesting. The error of measurement is the standard deviation of the difference between the true score and the obtained scores. The error of measurement allows the examiner to develop "confidence bands" that indicate a range of scores within which the individual's true score will fall a given percentage of time.

Fine Motor Movements using hands and fingers for tasks requiring precision.

Gross Motor Movements requiring the whole body for appropriate execution. Transfer of body weight and postural adjustment is involved.

Hyperactivity Excessive motor activity, manifested as excessive running or climbing, difficulty sitting still, or excessive movement in sleep.

IEP Individualized Educational Plan. A written outline of instructional and therapeutic strategies that will be used for the remediation of a handicapped student in special education.

IFSP Individualized Family Service Plan. A written outline of instructional and therapeutic strategies necessary to meet the preschool-age child's (birth to three years) and family's needs. Developed from child and family assessments conducted by a multidisciplinary team and with the family's input.

Interdisciplinary Format of shared communication, trust, openness, respect, and interdependence between professionals in establishing a diagnosis or developing prescriptive plans.

Learning Disability Condition whereby an individual's academic achievement level (in any specific academic area) is significantly below the level that would be predicted from the level of intellectual ability.

Minimal Brain Dysfunction (MBD) Subtle brain dysfunction in which a child exhibits a mixture of some or all of the following: learning disabilities, language disabilities, other inconsistencies among various cognitive functions, attention deficit disorder, gross, fine, and oral motor dyscoordinations.

Neurodevelopmental Examination Examination of the level of development in motor (gross and fine), language (expressive and receptive), visual problem solving, and social adaptive functioning.

Neurodevelopmental History History of the temporal sequence of development in motor (gross and fine), language (expressive and receptive), visual problem solving, and social adaptive functioning.

Norm-Referenced Test A test designed to determine how well the child performs on a particular task, in comparison with peers.

Norms Test scores based on the performance of a representative cross-section of students, usually a national sample.

Perceptual-Motor Integration The ability to integrate information from sensory channels (e.g., vision, touch, body position) with fine motor skills to achieve the desired outcome.

P. L. 94-142 The Education for All Handicapped Children Act of 1975, which provides for free appropriate education of all children who are handicapped, including children who are learning disabled, in the least restrictive educational environment.

P. L. 98-524 The Carl D. Perkins Vocational Education Act of 1984, enables students who are handicapped and disadvantaged to access the full range of vocational programs available to individuals who are not handicapped.

P. L. 99-457 Education of the Handicapped Amendments of 1986, which provides new incentives for the development of services to young children who are handicapped and their families. Stipulates development of an Individualized Family Service Plan (IFSP).

Primary Handicapping Conditions Handicapping conditions that have a neurological basis, including learning disabilities, speech-language disabilities, gross and fine motor dyscoordination, and attention-deficit hyperactivity disorder.

Regression Toward the Mean A statistical phenomenon whereby students who score higher or lower than the mean on a given test will be expected to score nearer the mean on a subsequent test. Regression toward the mean increases as the correlation between the two tests decreases.

Reliability The extent to which a test consistently measures what it measures. This includes consistency over time (test-retest reliability), and consistency across forms of the test (alternate form reliability), or consistency within the test items themselves (internal reliability).

Secondary Handicapping Conditions Handicapping conditions that do not have a direct neurological basis, but are the result of primary (neurologically based) conditions that have not been properly managed. The most common are poor self-concept and inappropriate attention-seeking behaviors.

Sensory Integration The ability to perceive discrete stimuli and to combine them into a meaningful whole generating an appropriate response.

Sensory Integrative Therapy Treatment involving sensory stimulation (vestibular, proprioceptive, and tactile) with the goal of improving the way a child processes and organizes sensations.

Slow Learner Term used to describe the child whose learning ability in all areas is delayed in comparison to children of the same chronological age. These children are characterized by low-normal to borderline intelligence, with corresponding slow academic achievement.

Soft Neurological Signs Neurological findings that are on a developmental continuum, that is, they appear and disappear with development and maturation of the nervous system. Pathology equates with the extent of their presence and the timing of their appearance and disappearance. Mirror movements and synkinesis represent the most commonly encountered.

Standard Score A type of test score that indicates how far an individual's performance deviates from the mean of the standardization sample (the representative sample from which the standard scores were derived). Standard scores for most tests have a mean of 100 and a standard deviation of 15.

Synkinesis Overflow or overshooting of muscle movements into surrounding muscle groups when a request is made for movement of an isolated muscle group.

Validity The extent to which a test actually measures what it purports to measure. A test's validity is determined by how well it samples from the domain of behaviors it was designed to measure (content validity), how well the test correlates with other measures of the same or similar construct (concurrent validity), how well the test predicts the child's future performance (predictive validity), and how helpful the test is in understanding the construct measured (construct validity).

Vestibular System The sensory system that responds to the position of the head in relation to gravity and accelerated or decelerated movement.

Word-Attack Skills A child's ability to decode unknown words, based on application of phonic skills (making grapheme-phoneme equivalences) and structural analysis skills (identifying word "parts," including root words, suffixes, and prefixes).

APPENDIX A

Parent Interview Form

Child's Name _____

Interviewee _____

1. Primary concerns: _____
2. Source of referral: _____
3. Current grade: _____
   school: _____
   teacher: _____
   special education services: _____
   type of class: _____
4. School history:
   preschool?

Grade	School	Services	Repeated?	Problems
K	_____	_____	_____	_____
1	_____	_____	_____	_____
2	_____	_____	_____	_____
3	_____	_____	_____	_____
4	_____	_____	_____	_____
5	_____	_____	_____	_____
6	_____	_____	_____	_____
7	_____	_____	_____	_____
8	_____	_____	_____	_____
9	_____	_____	_____	_____

5. Current school grades: _____
6. Teachers' complaints: _____ hyperactive
   _____ distractible
   _____ short attention span
   _____ won't stay in seat
   _____ shy/withdrawn
   _____ sloppy/disorganized
   _____ frustrated easily
   _____ talks out of turn
   _____ fails to complete assignments

_____ destructive
_____ disruptive
7. Specific weaknesses: _____ reading
_____ arithmetic
_____ spelling
_____ handwriting
_____ speech
_____ fine motor skills
_____ gross motor skills
_____ hearing/vision
8. Family: _____ father _____ mother _____ brothers (ages: ____)
_____ sisters (ages: _____) _____ other:
parents separated? _____ how long? _____
contact with noncustodial parent? _____
9. Language other than English at home? _____
10. Behavior problems at home?
_____ fails to listen to and follow instructions
_____ refuses to obey
_____ temper tantrums
_____ lies
_____ steals
_____ other
11. Chores required? _____
type? _____
problems? _____
12. Homework:
How much time spent each night? _____
How much time should be spent? _____
Supervision required? _____
Problems? _____
13. Many friends? _____
Interaction with peers? _____
14. Relationship with siblings? _____
15. Extracurricular activities: _____
What does the child like to do? _____
Organized teams/groups? _____

PARENT INTERVIEW FORM

16. Any unusual fears? _____
    Sleeping problems? _____
    Eating problems? _____
    Separation problems? _____
17. Self-concept? _____
18. Previous Testing? _____
19. Family history of learning problems?
    Mother: _____
    Father: _____
    Siblings: _____
    Other family members: _____
20. Medication for attention deficit disorder?
    Started:_____   Stopped:_____
    Current dosage: _____
    Schooldays/evenings/weekends/summers: _____
    Effectiveness: _____
    Problems: _____
    On medication today? _____ Time taken: _____
    Any other medications/health issues that might affect testing? _____
    _____

21. Other concerns? _____
    _____
    _____

APPENDIX B

TRANSITION RESOURCE LIST

COLLEGE/POSTSECONDARY TRAINING LD GUIDES

College Guide for Students with Learning Disabilities
J. Scalfani and M. J. Lynch
SPEDCO Associates
Farmingville, NY 11738

College Programs for Learning Disabled Students
National Association of College Admissions Counselors
Skokie, IL 60076

A Guide to Colleges for Learning Disabled Students
M. Liscio
Academic Press
Orlando, FL 32887

A Guide to Post-Secondary Educational Opportunities for the Learning Disabled
Time Out to Enjoy
Oak Park, IL 60303

LDA College List
Learning Disabilities Association of America
Pittsburgh, PA 15234

Learning Disabilities, Graduate School, and Careers
Pamela B. Adelman and Carol T. Wren
Learning Opportunities Program
Barat College
Lake Forest, IL 60045

Lovejoy's College Guide for the Learning Disabled
C. T. Straughn
Monarch Press
New York, NY 10001

McGuire-Shaw Postsecondary Selection Guide for Learning Disabled
  College Students
Special Education Center Publications
The University of Connecticut
Storrs, CT 06269

A National Directory of Four Year Colleges, Two Year Colleges and Post High School
  Training Programs for Young People with Learning Disabilities
P. M. Fielding, Editor
Partners in Publishing
Tulsa, OK 74127

Peterson's Guide to Colleges with Programs for Learning Disabled Students
C. T. Mangrum and S. S. Strichart, Editors
Peterson's Guides
Princeton, NJ 08540

TRANSITION RESOURCE LIST

ORGANIZATIONS/AGENCIES

Association on Handicapped Student Services Programs in
 Postsecondary Education
P. O. Box 21192
Columbus, OH 43221

College Handicapped and Exceptional Learners Programs and Services
Partners in Publishing
1419 East 1st Street
Tulsa, OK 74127

Council for Learning Disabilities
P. O. Box 40303
Overland Park, KS 66204

Division for Learning Disabilities
Council for Exceptional Children
1920 Association Drive
Reston, VA 22091

HEATH Resource Center
National Clearinghouse on Postsecondary Education for Individuals
 with Disabilities
Publisher of Information from HEATH, a newsletter published three times a year.
 (Subscription is free.)
One Dupont Circle
Washington, DC 20036

Learning Disability Association of America (formerly ACLD)
4156 Library Road
Pittsburgh, PA 15234

The National Center for Research on Vocational Education
The Ohio State University
1960 Kenny Road
Columbus, OH 43210

National Clearinghouse of Rehabilitation Training Materials
Oklahoma State University
115 USDA Building
Stillwater, OK 74078

National Information Center for Handicapped Children and Youths
P. O. Box 149
National Resource Center for Materials on Work Evaluation and Work Adjustment
Materials Development Center
University of Wisconsin-Stout
Menomonie, WI 54751

REFERENCES

Achenbach, T. M., Edelbrock, C. S., & Howell, C. T. (1987). Empirically-based assessment of the behavioral/emotional problems of 2–3-year-old children. *Journal of Abnormal Child Psychology, 15,* 629–650.

American Psychiatric Association. (1980). *Diagnostic and statistical manual of mental disorders* (3rd Ed.). Washington, DC: Author.

American Psychiatric Association. (1987). *Diagnostic and statistical manual of mental disorders* (3rd Ed.-Revised). Washington, DC: Author.

Applebee, A. (1978). *The child's concept of story.* Chicago: University of Chicago Press.

Arendt, R., MacLean, W., Jr., & Baumeister, A. (1988). Critique of sensory integration therapy and its application in mental retardation. *American Journal of Mental Retardation, 92*(5), 401–411.

Aylward, E. (1991). *Understanding children's testing.* Austin, TX: Pro-Ed.

Ayres, A. (1972a). Improving academic scores through sensory integration. *Journal of Learning Disabilities, 5*(6), 338–343.

Ayres, A. (1972b). *Sensory integration and learning disorders.* Los Angeles: Western Psychological Services.

Ayres, A. (1976). *The effect of sensory integrative therapy on learning disabled children: The final report of a research project.* Los Angeles: Center for the Study of Sensory Integrative Dysfunction.

Ayres, A. (1977). Effect of sensory integrative therapy on the coordination of children with choreoathetoid movements. *American Journal of Occupational Therapy, 31*(5), 291–293.

Ayres, A. (1980). *Sensory integration and the child.* Los Angeles: Western Psychological Services.

Ayres, A. (1989). *Sensory integration and praxis tests.* Los Angeles: Western Psychological Services.

Ayres, A., & Mailloux, Z. (1981). Influence of sensory integration procedures on language development. *American Journal of Occupational Therapy, 35*(6), 383–390.

Ayres, A., & Tickle, L. (1980). Hyper-responsivity to touch and vestibular stimuli as a predictor of positive response to sensory integration procedures in autistic children. *American Journal of Occupational Therapy, 34*(6), 375–381.

Bayley, N. (1969). *The Bayley scales of infant development.* New York: The Psychological Corporation.

Behar, L., & Stringfield, S. (1974). *The preschool behavior questionnaire.* Chapel Hill: University of North Carolina.

Bender, L. (1957). Specific reading disability as a maturational lag. *Bulletin of the Orton Society, 7,* 9–18.

Berk, R. (1984). *Screening and diagnosis of children with learning disabilities.* Springfield, IL: Charles C. Thomas.

Berruta-Clement, J. R., Schweinhart, L. J., Barnett, W. S., Epstein, A. S., & Weikart, D. P. (1984). *Changed lines: The effects of the Perry preschool project through age 19.* Ypsilanti, MI: High/Scope.

Blankenship, C., & Lilly, M. S. (1981). *Mainstreaming students with learning and behavior problems: Techniques for the classroom teacher.* New York: Holt, Rinehart, and Winston.

REFERENCES

Bowerman, M. (1976). Semantic factors in the acquisition of rules for word use and sentence construction. In D. M. Morehead and A. E. Morehead (Eds.), *Normal and deficient child language.* Baltimore, MD: University Park Press.

Bradley, C. (1937). The behavior of children receiving benzedrine. *American Journal of Psychiatry, 94,* 577–585.

Brown, A. L., & Campione, J. (1986). Psychological theory and the study of learning disabilities. *American Psychologist, 41,* 1059–1068.

Bryan, T., Donahue, M., & Pearl, R. (1981). Studies of learning disabled children's pragmatic competence. *Topics in Learning and Learning Disabilities, 1*(2), 29–39.

Budoff, M. (1987). The validity of learning potential assessment. In C. S. Lidz (Ed.), *Dynamic assessment an interactional approach* (pp. 52–81). New York: Guilford Press.

Cable, B. (1981). *A study of play behavior in learning disabled and normal preschool boys.* Unpublished doctoral dissertation, Northwestern University, Evanston, IL.

Camp, B., Blom, G., Herbert, F., & Van Doornenck, W. (1977). "Think aloud": A program for developing self-control in young aggressive boys. *Journal of Abnormal Child Psychology, 5,* 157–169.

Campbell, D., & Stanley, J. (1963). *Experimental and quasi-experimental designs for research.* Chicago: Rand McNally.

Campbell, S. B., Szumowski, E. K., Ewing, L. J., Gluck, D. S., & Breaux, A. M. (1982). A multidimensional assessment of parent-identified behavior problem toddlers. *Journal of Abnormal Child Psychology, 10*(4), 569–592.

Campione, J. (1989). Assisted assessment: A taxonomy of approaches and an outline of strengths and weaknesses. *Journal of Learning Disabilities, 22,* 151–165.

Carlson, J. S., & Weidl, K. H. (1979). Toward a differential testing approach: Testing the limits employing the Raven's matrices. *Intelligence, 3,* 323–344.

Carnine, D. (1979). Direct instruction: A successful system for educationally high-risk children. *Journal of Curriculum Studies, 11,* 29–45.

Casto, G., & Mastropieri, M. (1986). The efficacy of early intervention programs with handicapped children: A meta-analysis. *Exceptional Children, 52,* 417–424.

Cermak, S. (1985). Developmental dyspraxia. In E. A. Roy (Ed.), *Neuropsychological studies of apraxia and related disorders* (pp. 225–248). New York: Elsevier Science Publishers.

Cicci, R. L. (1978). *A study of pretended use of objects and graphic-pictorial representation in language impaired and normal preschool children.* Unpublished doctoral dissertation, Northwestern University, Evanston, IL.

Clark, F., Mailloux, Z., & Parham, D. (1989). *Sensory integration and children with learning disabilities* (2nd Ed.). St. Louis, MO: The C. V. Mosby Company.

Cone, T. E., & Wilson, L. R. (1981). Quantifying a severe discrepancy: A critical analysis. *Learning Disabilities Quarterly, 4*(4), 359–371.

Conners, C. K. (1973). Rating scales for use in drug studies with children. *Psychopharmacology bulletin* [special issue: *Pharmacotherapy with children*], 24–81.

Critchley, M. (1970). *The dyslexic child.* Springfield, IL: Charles Thomas.

Delaney, E., & Hopkins, T. (1987). *The Stanford-Binet intelligence scale: Fourth edition. Examiner's handbook.* Chicago: Riverside.

Deno, E. (1973). Special education as developmental capital. *Exceptional Children, 39*, 495.

Deno, E., & Fuchs, L. (1987). Developing a curriculum-based measurement systems for data-based special education problem solving. *Focus on Exceptional Children, 19*(6), 1–16.

Doll, E. J. (1990). Review of the Kaufman Test of Educational Achievement. *The tenth mental measurement yearbook.* Lincoln, NB: University of Nebraska Press.

Donnelly, M., Zametkin, A. J., Rapoport, J. L., Ismond, D. R., Weingartner, H., Lane, E., Oliver, J., Linnoila, M. D., & Potter, W. Z. (1986). Treatment of childhood hyperactivity with desipramine: Plasma drug concentration, cardiovascular effects, plasma and urinary catecholamine levels, and clinical response. *Clinical Pharmacological Therapy, 39*, 72–81.

Dreisbach, M., & Keogh, B. K. (1982). Testwiseness as a factor in readiness test performance of young Mexican-American children. *Journal of Educational Psychology, 74*(2), 224–229.

Dunn, W. (1988). Basic and applied neuroscience research provides a basis for sensory integration theory. *American Journal of Mental Retardation, 92*(5), 420–422.

Dunn, W. (1991a). *Pediatric occupational therapy: Facilitating effective service provision.* Thorofare, NJ: Slack.

Dunn, W. (1991b). Integrated related services. In L. H. Meyer, C. A. Peck, & L. Brown (Eds.), *Critical issues in the lives of people with severe disabilities* (pp. 353–377). Baltimore, MD: Paul H. Brookes.

Dunn, W., & Campbell, P. (1991). Designing pediatric service provision. In W. Dunn (Ed.), *Pediatric occupational therapy: Facilitating effective service provision* (pp. 139–159). Thorofare, NJ: Slack.

Dunn, W., Campbell, P., Oetter, P., Hall, S., Berger, E., & Strickland, L. (1989). *Guidelines for occupational therapy services in early intervention and preschool services.* Rockville, MD: The American Occupational Therapy Association.

Elksnin, L. K., & Elksnin, N. (1990). Using collaborative consultation with parents to promote effective vocational programming. *Career Development for Exceptional Individuals, 13*, 135–142.

Feichtner, S.H. (1989). *School-to-work transition for at-risk youth* (Information Series No. 339). Columbus: The Ohio State University, ERIC Clearinghouse on Adult, Career, and Vocational Education, Center on Education and Training for Employment.

Feuerstein, R. (1979). *The dynamic assessment of retarded performers: The learning potential assessment device; theory, instruments, and techniques.* Baltimore, MD: University Park Press.

REFERENCES

Friedman, J. (1984). *Classification skills in normally hearing/achieving, oral deaf, and language impaired preschoolers: A study in language and conceptual thought.* Unpublished doctoral dissertation, Northwestern University, Evanston, IL.

Gandara, P., Keogh, B. K., & Yoshioka-Maxwell, B. (1980). Predicting academic performance of Anglo and Mexican-American kindergarten children. *Psychology in the Schools, 17,* 174–177.

Gersten, R. (1985). Direct instruction with special education students: A review of evaluation research. *Journal of Special Education, 19,* 41–58.

Gesell, A., & Amatruda, C. S. (1947). *Developmental diagnosis: Normal and abnormal child development: Clinical methods and pediatric applications.* New York: Paul B. Hoeber.

Gresham, F. M. (1990). Best practices in social skills training. In A. Thomas and J. Grimes (Eds.), *Best practices in school psychology-II* (pp. 695–709). Washington, DC: National Association of School Psychologists.

Guerin, G. R., & Maier, A. S. (1983). *Informal assessment in education.* Palo Alto, CA: Mayfield Publishing.

Halliday, M. (1975). *Learning how to mean: Explorations in the development of language.* (pp. 9–21). London: Edward Arnold.

Halpern, J. M., Gittleman, R., & Klein, D. F. (1984). Reading disabled hyperactive children: A distinct subgroup of attention deficit disorder with hyperactivity? *Journal of Abnormal Child Psychology, 12,* 1–14.

Harrington, R. (1984). Assessment of learning disabled children. In S. J. Weaver (Ed.), *Testing children.* Kansas City, MO: Test Corporation of America.

Hecht, B.F. (1986). Problems in language development. In B. K. Keogh (Ed.), *Advances in Special Education: Developmental Problems in Infancy and the Preschool Years.* Greenwich, CT: JAI Press.

Hedrick, D., Prather, E., & Tobin, A. (1975). *Sequenced inventory of communication development.* Seattle: University of Washington Press.

Heshusius, L. (1991). Curriculum-based assessment and direct instruction: Critical reflections on fundamental assumptions. *Exceptional children, 57,* 315–328.

Hinshelwood, J. (1917). *Congenital word-blindness.* London: Lewis.

Horn, W. F., & Packard, T. (1986). Early identification of learning problems: A meta-analysis. *Journal of Educational Psychology, 77,* 557–607.

Howell, K., & Moorehead, M. K. (1987). *Curriculum-based evaluation for special and remedial education.* Columbus, OH: Merrill.

Idol, L., Paolucci-Whitcomb, P., & Nevin, A. (1986). *Collaborative consultation.* Rockville, MD: Aspen.

Interagency Committee on Learning Disabilities (1987). *Learning Disabilities. A Report to Congress.*

Johnson, C. (1981). *The diagnosis of learning disabilities.* Boulder, CO: Pruett Publishing.

Johnson, D. J. (1983). Design for individualization of language intervention programs. In J. Miller, D. E. Yoder, & R. Schiefelbusch

(Eds.), *Contemporary issues in language intervention.* Rockville, MD: The American Speech-Language-Hearing Association.

Kamhi, A., Catts, H., Koenig, L., & Lewis, B. (1984). Hypothesis-testing and nonlinguistic symbolic activities in language-impaired children. *Journal of Speech and Hearing Disorders, 49,* 169–176.

Kaufman, A. (1976a). Verbal-Performance IQ discrepancies on the WISC-R. *Journal of Consulting and Clinical Psychology, 44,* 739–744.

Kaufman, A. (1976b). A new approach to the interpretation of test scatter on the WISC-R. *Journal of Learning Disabilities, 9,* 160–168.

Kaufman, A. (1979). *Intelligent testing with the WISC-R.* New York: John Wiley & Sons.

Kaufman, A. (1983). Some questions and answers about the Kaufman Assessment Battery for Children (K-ABC). *Journal of Psycho-educational Assessment, 4,* 205–218.

Kaufman, A., & Doppelt, J. (1976). Analysis of WISC-R standardization data in terms of the stratification variables. *Child Development, 47,* 165–171.

Kaufman, A., & Kaufman, N. (1983). *Kaufman Assessment Battery for Children Interpretive Manual.* Circle Pines, MN: American Guidance Service.

Kendall, P., & Finch, A. (1979). Developing nonimpulsive behavior in children: Cognitive-behavioral strategies for self-control. In P. Kendall & S. Hollon (Eds.), *Cognitive-behavioral interventions: Theory, research, and procedures.* New York: Plenum Press.

Keogh, B. K., Major-Kingsley, S., Omori-Gordon, H., & Reid, H. P. (1982). *A Marker System for the Field of Learning Disabilities.* Syracuse, NY: Syracuse University Press.

Kinsbourne, M. (1975). The ontogeny of cerebral dominance. *Annals of the New York Academy of Sciences, 263,* 244–250.

Knickerbocker, B. (1980). *A holistic approach to the treatment of learning disorders.* Thorofare, NJ: Charles B. Slack.

Larrivee, B. (1989). Effective strategies for academically handicapped students in the regular classroom. In R. E. Slavin, N. L. Karweit, & N. A. Madden (Eds.), *Effective programs for students at risk* (pp. 291–319). Boston: Allyn & Bacon.

Lazar, I., & Darlington, R. (1982). Lasting effects of early education: A report from the consortium for longitudinal studies. *SRCD Monograph, 46*(2–3). Serial No. 195.

Lazarus, B. D., McKenna, M. C., & Lynch, D. (1989/1990). Peabody Individual Achievement Test-Revised (PIAT-R). *Diagnostique, 15,* 135–148.

Leigh, J. (1986). NJCLD position paper: Learning disabilities and the preschool-child. *Learning Disability Quarterly, 9,* 158–163.

Levine, M., Brooks, R., & Shonkoff, J. (1980). *A pediatric approach to learning disorders.* New York: John Wiley & Sons.

Lidz, C. S. (1987). *Dynamic assessment: An interactional approach to evaluation learning potential.* New York: Guilford Press.

Mastropieri, M. A. (1988). Learning disabilities in early childhood. In K. A. Kavale (Ed.), *Learning Disabilities: State of Art and Practice.* Boston: Little, Brown.

McCarthy, D. (1972). *McCarthy scales of children's abilities.* San Antonio, TX: The Psychological Corporation.

McCarthy, J. (1989). Through my kaleidoscope-1989. Elements from the past with promise for their future. *Learning Disabilities Focus, 4*(2), 67–72.

McKeever, W., & VanDeventer, A. (1975). Dyslexic adolescents: Evidence of impaired visual and auditory language processing associated with normal lateralization and visual responsivity. *Cortex, 11,* 361–378.

McLeod, J. (1979). Educational underachievement: Toward a defensible psychometric definition. *Journal of Learning Disabilities, 12,* 322–330.

Mitchell, J. V., Jr. (1985). *The Ninth Mental Measurements Yearbook.* Lincoln, NE: The Buros Mental Measurement Institute.

Montgomery, P., & Richter, E. (1977). Effect of sensory integrative therapy on the neuromotor development of retarded children. *Physical Therapy, 57,* 799–806.

National Joint Committee for Learning Disabilities. (1981). *Learning disabilities: Issues on definition.* Unpublished position paper. (Available from Drake Duane, NJCLD Chairperson, c/o The Orton Dyslexia Society, 8415 Bellona Lane, Towson, MD 21204).

Ness, J. E. (1989). The high jump: Transition issues of learning disabled students and their parents. *Academic Therapy, 25,* 33–40.

Newborg, J., Stock, J., Wnek, L., Guidubaldi, J., & Svinicki, J. (1984). *Battelle developmental inventory.* Allen, TX: DLM Teaching Resources.

Ottenbacher, K. (1982). Sensory integration therapy: Affect or effect. *American Journal of Occupational Therapy, 36*(9), 571–578.

Patton, J. R., & Polloway, E. A. (1987). Analyzing college courses. *Academic Therapy, 22,* 273–280.

Pressley, M. (1990). *Cognitive stategy instruction that really improves children's academic performance.* Cambridge, MA: Brookline Books.

Public Law 94–142. (1975). Education for All Handicapped Children Act.

Public Law 98–524. (1984). Carl D. Perkins Vocational Education Act.

Public Law 99–457. (1986). Education for the Handicapped Amendments.

Rapoport, J. L., Zametkin, A., Donnelly, M., & Ismond, D. (1985). New drug trials in attention deficit disorder. *Psychopharmacology Bulletin, 21,* 232–236.

Reeve, R. C. (Ed.). (1989–1990). Monograph: Assessment for the 1990s—Critical Reviews of Recent Instruments. *Diagnostique, 15,* 1–4.

Reid, D. K., & Stone, C. A. (1991). Why is cognitive instruction effective? Underlying learning mechanisms. *Remedial and Special Education, 12*(3), 8–19.

Reynell, J. (1979). *Reynell-Zinkin Scales: Developmental scales for young visually handicapped children.* Windsor, England: NFER Publishers.

Reynolds, C. (1984). Critical measurement issues in learning disabilities. *Journal of Special Education, 18*(4), 451–476.

Safer, D., & Allen, R. (1976). *Hyperactive children: Diagnosis and management.* Baltimore, MD: University Park Press.

Salvia, J., & Hughes, C. (1990). *Curriculum-based assessment: Testing what is taught.* New York: Macmillan.

Scarborough, H. (1990). Very early language deficits in dyslexic children. *Child Development, 61*(6), 1728–1743.

Schumaker, J. B., Deshler D. D., Alley, G. R., & Warner, M. M. (1983). Toward the development of an intervention model for learning disabled adolescents: The University of Kansas Institute. *Exceptional Education Quarterly, 4,* 45–74.

Sebrechts, M. M., Shaywitz, S. E., Shaywitz, B. A., Jatlow, P., Anderson, G. M., & Cohen, D. J. (1986). Components of attention, methylphenidate dosage, and blood levels in children with attention deficit disorder. *Pediatrics, 77,* 222–227.

Siperstein, G. N. (1988). Students with learning disabilities in college: The need for a programmatic approach to critical transitions. *Journal of Learning Disabilities, 21,* 431–436.

Sitlington, P. L. (1986). *Transition, special needs, and vocational education.* Columbus, OH: The National Center for Research in Vocational Education, The Ohio State University.

Sitlington, P. L., & Frank, A. R. (1990). Are adolescents with learning disabilities successfully crossing the bridge into adult life? *Learning Disability Quarterly, 13,* 97–111.

Sixth Annual Report to Congress on the Implementation of Public Law 94–142: The Education of All Handicapped Children Act (1984). Office of Special Education, U.S. Department of Education.

Stake, R., & Wardrop, J. (1971). Gain score errors in performance contracting. *Research in the Teaching of English, 5,* 226–229.

Stein, N., & Glenn, C. (1979). An analysis of story comprehension in elementary school children. In R. O. Freedle (Ed.), *New directions in discourse processing: Advances in discourse processes* (p. 9) Norwood, NJ: Ablex.

Strichart, S. S., & Mangrum, C. T. II (1985). Selecting a college for the LD student. *Academic Therapy, 20,* 475–479.

Sugai, G. (1985). Recording classroom events: Maintaining a critical incidents log. *Teaching exceptional children,* Winter, 1986, 98–102.

Thorndike, R. (1963). *The concept of over and underachievement.* New York: Columbia University Press.

Thorndike, R., Hagen, E., & Sattler, J. (1986). *Stanford-Binet intelligence scale (4th Ed.): Technical manual.* Chicago: Riverside.

Ullmann, R. K., Sleator, E. K., & Sprague, R. L. (1985). A change in mind: The Conners Abbreviated Rating Scales reconsidered. *Journal of Abnormal Child Psychology, 13,* 553–565.

U.S. Office of Education. (1977). Assistance to states for education for handicapped children: Procedures for evaluating specific learning disabilities. *Federal Register, 42*(250), 62082–62085.

Van Reusen, A. K., Bos, C. S., Schumaker, J. B., & Deshler, D. D. (1987). *The education planning strategy.* Lawrence, KS: EXCELLenterprises.

Vogel, S. (1974). Syntactic abilities in normal and dyslexic children. *Journal of Learning Disabilities, 7,* 47–53.

Wagner, M. (1989, March). *The transition experiences of youth with disabilities: A report from the national longitudinal transition study.* Paper presented at the meeting of the Division for Research, Council for Exceptional Children, San Francisco, CA.

Wechsler, D. (1989). *Manual for the Wechsler Preschool and Primary Scale of Intelligence.* San Antonio, TX: The Psychological Corp.

Wiig, E., & Semel, E. (1984). *Language assessment and intervention for the learning disabled,* (2nd Ed). Columbus OH: Charles E. Merrill.

Witelson, S. (1977). Neural and cognitive correlates of developmental dyslexia: Age and sex differences. In C. Shagaes, S. Gershon, & A. Friedhoff (Eds.), *Psychopathology and brain dysfunction.* New York: Raven Press.

Wren, C. (1980). *The relationship of auditory and cognitive processes to syntactic patterns of learning disabled and normal children.* Unpublished doctoral dissertation, Northwestern University, Evanston, IL.

REFERENCE LIST OF TESTS

Tests included in this list are not necessarily endorsed by the authors. A number of these tests are discussed in the text and are referenced in the index.

ACTeRS (1988)
MetriTech, Inc.

Analytic Reading Inventory (1989)
M. L. Woods and A. J. Moe
Psychological Corporation
555 Academic Ct., San Antonio,
  TX 78204

Basic Achievement Skills Individual Screener (BASIS) (1982)
Psychological Corporation
555 Academic Ct., San Antonio,
  TX 78204

Battelle Developmental Inventory (1984)
DLM Teaching Resources
One DLM Park, P. O. Box 4000, Allen,
  TX 75002

Bayley Scales of Infant Development (1969)
Psychological Corporation
7500 Old Oak Blvd., Cleveland,
  OH 44130

Behavior Evaluation Scale—2 (BES-2) (1990)
S. B. McCarney and J. E. Leigh
Hawthorne Educational Services
P. O. Box 7540, Columbia, MO 65205

Behavior Problem Checklist— Revised (1983)
H. C. Quay
P. O. Box 248074
University of Miami, Coral Gables,
  FL 32124

Behavior Rating Profile (1983)
L. L. Brown and D. D. Hammill
PRO-ED
Austin, TX 78735

Bender Visual Motor Gestalt Test (1946)
Lauretta Bender
American Orthopsychiatric Association
49 Sheridan Ave., Albany, NY 12210

Benton Revised Visual Retention Test (1974)
Arthur Benton
The Psychological Corporation
555 Academic Ct., San Antonio,
  TX 78204

Brigance Diagnostic Inventory of Basic Skills (1977)

Brigance Diagnostic Inventory of Early Development (1978)

Brigance Diagnostic Inventory of Essential Skills (1980)

Brigance Preschool Screen (1985)
Albert H. Brigance
Curriculum Associates, Inc.
5 Esquire Rd., North Billerica,
  MA 01862-2589

Bruininks–Oseretsky Test of Motor Proficiency (1978)
Robert H. Bruininks
American Guidance Service
Publishers Building, Circle Pines,
  MN 55014

California Achievement Tests (1977, 1978)
CTB-McGraw-Hill
2500 Garden Rd., Monterey, CA 93940

Child Behavior Checklist & Youth Self Report Teacher Report Form (1986)
T. M. Achenbach and C. S. Edelbrock
Department of Psychiatry
University of Vermont
Burlington, VT 05405

REFERENCE LIST OF TESTS

Children's Apperception Test (1980)
Leopold Bellak and Sonya Sorel Bellak
C. P. S., Inc.
Box 83, Larchmont, NY 10538

Classroom Reading Inventory (1986)
M. J. Silvaroli and W. C. Brown Co.
2460 Kerper Blvd., Dubuque, IA 52001

Cognitive Abilities Test (1983)
Robert L. Thorndike and
 Elizabeth Hagen
Riverside Publishing Co.
8420 Bryn Mawr Ave., Chicago, IL 60631

**Cognitive Skills Assessment Battery,
 Second Edition (1981)**
Teachers College Press
P. O. Box 1540, Hagerstown, MD 21740

**Comprehensive Test of Basic Skills
 (1981, 1982, 1983)**
CTB-McGraw-Hill
Del Monte Research Park
2500 Garden Road, Monterey, CA 93940

**Curriculum Referenced Tests of
 Mastery (1983, 1984)**
Psychological Corporation
555 Academic Ct., San Antonio, TX 78204

**Detroit Tests of Learning
 Aptitude (1975)**
Harry J. Baker and Bernice Leland
Bobbs-Merrill Educational Publishing
4300 West 62nd St., P. O. Box 7080,
 Indianapolis, IN 46206

**Developmental Indicators for the
 Assessment of Learning—
 Revised (DIAL-R) (1983)**
Childcraft Education Corporation
20 Kilmer Road, P. O. Box 3081, Edison,
 NJ 08818-3081

**Developmental Test of Visual-Motor
 Integration, 3rd Revision (1989)**
Keith E. Beery and Norman A. Buktenica
Modern Curriculum Press, Inc.
13900 Prospect Road, Cleveland,
 OH 44136

**Diagnostic Reading Scales—
 Revised (1981)**
G. D. Spache
CTB Macmillan/McGraw-Hill
2500 Garden Road, Monterey, CA 93940

Dyadic Interaction Analysis (1969)
J. E. Brophy and T. L. Good
Research Development Center
University of Texas
Austin, TX 78712

Ekwall Reading Inventory (1979)
E. Ekwall
Allyn & Bacon
160 Gould Street, Needham Heights,
 MA 02194

**Frostig Developmental Test of Visual
 Perception (1961)**
Marianne Frostig and Associates
Consulting Psychologists Press, Inc.
577 College Avenue, P. O. Box 60070,
 Palo Alto, CA 94306

**Full Range Picture Vocabulary
 Test (1948)**
R. B. Ammons and H. S. Ammons
Psychological Test Specialists
Box 9229, Missoula, MT 59805

Gates–MacGinitie Reading Tests (1978)
The Riverside Publishing Company
8420 Bryn Mawr Ave, Chicago, IL 60632

**Gates–McKillop–Horowitz Reading
 Diagnostic Tests (1981)**
Teachers College Press
1234 Amsterdam Ave., New York,
 NY 10027

Gesell Developmental Schedules (1947)
Gesell, A. and Amatruda, C.
Developmental Diagnosis.
 New York: Hoeber

Gesell School Readiness Test (1980)
Programs for Education, Inc.,
 Department W83
82 Park Avenue, Flemington, NJ 08822

Goldman–Fristoe–Woodcock Auditory Skills Test Battery (1976)
Ronald Goldman, Macalyne Fristoe, and Richard W. Woodcock
American Guidance Service
Publisher's Building, Circle Pines, MN 55014

House–Tree–Person Technique (1981)
John N. Buck
Western Psychological Services
12031 Wilshire Boulevard, Los Angeles, CA 90025

Illinois Test of Psycholinguistic Abilities (1968)
Samuel A. Kirk, James J. McCarthy, and Winifred D. Kirk
University of Illinois Press
54 E. Gregory Dr., Box 5081, Station A., Champaign, IL 61820

Iowa Test of Basic Skills (ITBS) (1986)
A. N. Hieronymus, H. D. Hoover, and E. F. Lindquist
The Riverside Publishing Company
8420 Bryn Mawr Ave., Chicago, IL 60632

Kaufman Assessment Battery for Children (1983)
A. S. Kaufman and N. L. Kaufman
American Guidance Service
Publisher's Building, Circle Pines, MN 55014

Kaufman Test of Educational Achievement (KTEA) (1985)
A. S. Kaufman and N. L. Kaufman
American Guidance Service
Publisher's Building, Circle Pines, MN 55014

KeyMath–Revised (KMR) (1988)
A. J. Connolly
American Guidance Service
Publisher's Building, Circle Pines, MN 55014

McCarthy Scales of Children's Abilities (1972)
Dorothea McCarthy
The Psychological Corporation
555 Academic Ct, San Antonio, TX 78204-2498

Memory for Designs Test (1960)
Frances K. Graham and Barbara S. Kendall
Psychological Test Specialists
Box 9229, Missoula, MT 59807

Metropolitan Achievement Tests (MATS) (1984)
G. A. Prescott, I. H. Balow, T. R. Hogan, and R. C. Farr
The Psychological Corporation
555 Academic Ct., San Antonio, TX 78204

Minnesota Child Development Inventory (1974)
Behavior Science Systems, Inc.
P. O. Box 1108, Minneapolis, MN 55440

Motor-Free Visual Perception Test (1972)
Ronald R. Celarusso and Donald D. Hammill
Academic Therapy Publications
20 Commercial Boulevard, Novato, CA 94947

Multilevel Academic Survey Test (MAST) (1985)
K. W. Howell, S. H. Zucker, and M. K. Moorehead
The Psychological Corporation
555 Academic Ct., San Antonio, TX 78204

Otis-Lennon Mental Ability Test (1982)
Arthur S. Otis and Roger T. Lennon
The Psychological Corporation
555 Academic Ct., San Antonio, TX 78204

Peabody Individual Achievement Test—Revised (PIAT–R) (1989)
F. C. Markwardt, Jr.
American Guidance Service
Publisher's Building, Circle Pines, MN 55014

Peabody Picture Vocabulary Test—Revised (1981)
Lloyd M. Dunn and Leota M. Dunn
American Guidance Service
Publisher's Building, Circle Pines, MN 55014

Preschool Behavior Questionnaire (1974)
Journal of Abnormal Child Psychology, 5, 265-275.

Pupil Rating Scale Revised: Screening for Learning Disabilities (1981)
Grune & Stratton
111 Fifth Avenue, New York, NY 10003

Quick Test (1962)
R. B. Ammons and C. H. Ammons
Psychological Test Specialists
Box 9229, Missoula, MT 59807

Reynell Developmental Language Scales—Revised (1977)
NFER–Nelson Publishing Co.
Darville House, 2 Oxford Road East Windson Berkshire
SL4 1DF, England

Revised Behavior Problem Checklist (RBPC) (1987)
H. C. Quay and D. R. Peterson
P. O. Box 248074
University of Miami
Coral Gables, FL 33124

Rhode Island Profile of Early Learning Behavior (1982)
Jamestown Publishers
P. O. Box 6743, Providence RI 02940

Rorschach Psychodiagnostic Test (1981)
Hermann Rorschach
Hans Huber
Distributed by Grune & Stratton
111 Fifth Ave., New York, NY 10003

School Situation Questionnaire (1987)
R. A. Barkley and C. Edelbrock
In R. J. Prinz (Ed.) *Advances in behavioral assessment of children and families* (Vol. 3, pp. 157-176)
Greenwich, CT: JAI Press

Sequenced Inventory of Communication Development (SICD) (1979)
University of Washington Press
P. O. Box 85569, Seattle, WA 98105

Slingerland Pre-Reading Screening Procedures—Revised (1980)
Educators Publishing Service
75 Moulton Street, Cambridge, MA 02238-9101

Slosson Intelligence Test (1981)
Richard L. Slosson
Slosson Educational Publications, Inc.
P. O. Box 280, East Aurora, NY 14052

SRA Achievement Series (1978)
R. A. Naslund, L. P. Thrope, and D. W. LeFever
Science Research Associates
155 North Wacker Dr., Chicago, IL 60606

Stanford–Binet Intelligence Scale (1986)
R. L. Thorndike, E. P. Hagen, and J. M. Sattler
The Riverside Publishing Co.
8420 Bryn Mawr Ave., Chicago, IL 60631

Stanford Diagnostic Mathematics Test (1985)
L. S. Madden, E. R. Gardner, and C. S. Collins
The Psychological Corporation
555 Academic Ct., San Antonio, TX 78204

System to Plan Early Childhood Services (SPECS) (1991)
American Guidance Service
Publisher's Building, Circle Pines, MN 55014

Test of Early Language Development (TELD) (1981)

Test of Language Development— Primary (1982)
PRO-ED
Industrial Oaks Blvd., Austin, TX 78735

Test of Mathematical Abilities (TOMA) (1991)
V. L. Brown and E. McEntire
PRO-ED
8700 Shoal Creek Blvd., Austin, TX 78758

Thematic Apperception Test (1943)
Henry Alexander Murray
Harvard University Press
79 Garden Street, Cambridge, MA 02138

Utah Test of Language Development. Revised Edition (1978)
Communication Research
  Associates, Inc.
P. O. Box 11012, Salt Lake City, UT 84147

Wechsler Adult Intelligence Scale— Revised (1981)
Wechsler Intelligence Scale for Children—Revised (1974)

Wechsler (*continued*)

Wechsler Preschool and Primary Scale of Intelligence—Revised (1989)
David Wechsler
The Psychological Corporation
555 Academic Ct., San Antonio, TX 78204

Woodcock–Johnson Psycho- Educational Battery—Revised
R. W. Woodcock and M. B. Johnson
DLM Teaching Resources
One DLM Park, Allen, TX 75002

Subject Index

A

Academic achievement and intellectual abilities, identifying discrepancy between, 123–132
ADHD. *See* Attention-Deficit Hyperactivity Disorder
Adolescent with LD, transition for
    from high school to employment, 195–196
    legislation affecting efforts, 194–195
    roles of professionals and families, 196–198
    secondary program models, 192–193
Assessment for language, approaches to, 102–103
Attention-deficit hyperactivity disorder (ADHD), and preschool children, 24–25
    definition, 6–7, 9, 10
    educational evaluation of, 51
    identifying, 136–139
    and interdisciplinary process for LD, 12
Attention–deficit hyperactivity disorder (ADHD), planning for treatment
    environmental accommodations for management of, 170–175
        home-based, 173–175
        school-based, 171–173
    use of psychotropic medication
Attention–deficit hyperactivity disorder *(continued)*
        for management of, 175–179
    remediation, 169–170
Attentional, motivational, and behavioral problems, 120–121
Auditory memory, 54–55
Auditory processes, 105–109
    discrimination, 105–106
    memory, 107
    oral formulation of ideas, 109
    retrieval, 107–108
    sequencing, 108
    verbal comprehension, 106

B

Basic Skills Remediation Model for adolescents, 192
Bayley Scales of Infant Development, 20
Behavior problems
    managing, 182–188
    of preschool children, 25–26
    specific, identifying, 142–143
Behaviors to observe during intelligence testing, 68–72
Boehm Test of Basic Concepts, 30

C

Carl D. Perkins Vocational Act (Public Law 98-524), 3

Carl D. Perkins Vocational Act *(continued)*
    and adolescent with LD, 194–195
Clumsiness/incoordination, 118
Cognitive and psychosocial skills, problems with, 120–121
Cognitive development, assessing, 27–28
Cognitive-achievement comparison
    choosing measure of intelligence for, 128–130
    considering individual subtests scores in, 130–131
    flexibility in diagnosis, need for, 131–132
College, making transition to, 198–202
Compensatory model for adolescents, 193
Comprehensive Test of Basic Skills, 30
Criterion-referenced tests (CRT), 92–93
    definition of, 217
    strengths and limitations of, 94–95

D

Developmental Indicators for the Assessment of Learning — Revised (DIAL-R), 30
Diagnostic criteria, of preschool children, additional, 32–33
Diagnostic and Statistical Manual of Mental Disorders, third edition (DSM-III)
    and definition of ADHD, 6, 136–137
Direct assessment, 30–31
Discrepancy model for
    identification of, 27
    definition, 22–23
    cognitive development, assessing, 27–28
    rating scales, 29–30
    specific skills, assessing, 28–29
    test performances, influences of, 31–32

Discrimination, auditory, 105–106
Dynamic assessment, 95–96
Dyscalculia, 5
    definition of, 217
Dyseidetic dyslexics, 134
Dysgraphia, 5
Dyslexia, 5
    definition of, 217
Dysphonic dyslexics, 134
    definition of, 217

E

Education for all Handicapped Children Act, legislation affecting transition efforts of adolescent with LD, 194–195
Education for all Handicapped Children Act (Public Law 94-142), 1–2, 3
    and definition of learning disabilities, 1–2,
    eligibility definitions, 3
    and Public Law 99-457, 3, 6
    and treatment of LD, 147–148
Educational evaluation of LD
    assessment, 84–96
        curriculum-based assessment and measurement, 93–95
        limitations, 89
        measurement problems in establishing discrepancy, 89–92
        standardized achievement and diagnostic tests, 86–89
        standardized norm-referenced tests, 85
    differences with psychological evaluation, 83–84
        inventories, rating scales, checklists, 98–99
        observation, 97–98
Educational quotients (EQs), predicting, 127–128
    definition, 217
Emotional disturbance, secondary, managing, 188–190

SUBJECT INDEX

Emotional problems, identifying, 141–142
Employment, making transition from high school to, 195–196
Environmental accommodations for management of ADHD, 170–175
Error of measurement, definition, 217
Expectancy formulae, simple, 124–125

F

Families and professionals, role of in transition for adolescent with LD, 196–198
Family problems, identifying, 142
Fine motor, definition of, 217
Fine motor/visual motor integration, poor, 120
Functional communication, problems with, 115

G

Gesell drawings, and visual/perceptual development, 51–53
Gesell Developmental Schedules, 20
Grade level deviations, 124
Gross motor, definition, 218
Gross motor clumsiness, identifying, 140
Gross motor developmental milestones, 39

H

Handedness, laterally and dominance, 53–55
Handwriting slowness and inefficiency, identifying, 139–140
Handwriting disabilities, accommodations to circumvent LD, 166–167
Hard neurological signs, 55–56
Home, behavior management system in, 185
Hyperactivity, definition of, 217

I

Individualized College Plan (ICP), 199
Individualized Educational Plan (IEP)
    components of, 149–150
    considerations for developing, 152–153
    developmental team, 148
    implementation of, 151–152
Individualized Family Service Plan (IFSP)
    components of, 150–151
    developmental team, 149
Informal assessment, 96–99
Intellectual functioning tests, selection of, 61
Intelligence tests
    for older children, 67
    for preschool children, 66–67
Intelligence, choosing measure of, 128–130
Interdisciplinary diagnosis
    associated problems, identifying, 135–143
        ADHD, 136–139
        behavior problems, specific, 142–143
        emotional problems, 141–142
        family problems, 142
        gross motor clumsiness, 140
        language or speech problems, 140–141
        problems with organizational skills or study skills, 139
    discrepancy between academic achievement and intellectual abilities, identifying, 123–132
        educational quotients, predicting, 127–128
        grade level deviations, 124
        regression toward the mean, concept, 126–127
        simple expectancy formulae, 124–125
        standard scores, 125–126

Interdisciplinary diagnosis
(continued)
   preschool-age children at risk for LD, identifying, 132–134
   strengths and weaknesses in learning style, identifying, 134–135
Interdisciplinary process in diagnosis and treatment of LD
   definition, 11
   process, 11–15
Interdisciplinary team process, goal of, 205–213
   diagnoses presentation, 206–208
   follow-up, planning, 212–213
   parent's questions, answering, 210–212
      etiology discussion, 211
      prognosis discussion, 211–212
   therapeutic recommendations presentation, 208–210
IQ tests, 59–61

K

Kaufman Assessment Battery for children (K-ABC) test, 28, 61–66, 79, 130, 138
   simultaneous-sequential processing differences and subtest scatter, 75–76
Kaufman Test of Educational Achievement (KTEA), 86–87

L

Language evaluation of LD, 101–102
   assessment, approaches to, 102–103
   auditory processes, 105–109
      discrimination, 105–106
      memory, 107
      oral formulation of ideas, 109

Language evaluation of LD
(continued)
      retrieval, 107–108
      sequencing, 108
      verbal comprehension, 106
   rule systems, 103–105
Language functioning, 46–47
Language, expressive and receptive, 40
Language problems, of preschool children, 23–24
Language or speech problems, 140–141
Learning Strategies Curriculum, 193
Learning, generalization of, problems with, 121
Learning disabilities caused by primary handicapping conditions, 5–6
Learning disabilities
   definition of, 1–4, 9
   etiology of, 8–10
   interdisciplinary process of diagnosis and treatment, 11–15
   prevalence of, 8
   primary handicapping conditions, 4–7
   secondary handicapping conditions, 7
   slow learner, 8
Legislation affecting transition efforts of adolescent with LD, 194–195
Life tasks, problems with, 116

M

Mathematics disability, 5, 165
MBD. See Minimal brain dysfunction
McCarthy Scales of Children's Abilities, 28
Memory, auditory, 107
Methylphenidate, administration of, 177–178
Metropolitan Achievement Tests, 30–31
Minimal brain dysfunction (MBD), 7
   definition of, 218

SUBJECT INDEX

Minnesota Child Development Inventory, 20
Motor abilities, gross/fine/oral, assessment of, 47–48
Motor planning (dyspraxia), poor, 118
Multidisciplinary process in LD, comparison with interdisciplinary process, 11

N

National Joint Committee for Learning Disabilities (NJCLD), 2
Neurodevelopmental evaluation for the LD
    history and examination for school-age child, 48–56
    identification of preschool children at risk, 36–48
        examination, 43–56
        history, 36–42
Neurodevelopmental indicators, use of to identify LD in preschool children, 22, 26–27
Ninth Mental Measurement Yearbook, 28
Norm-referenced test, definition, 218

O

Occupational therapy evaluation
    interference with performance, underlying factors, 116–121
        problems with cognitive and psychosocial skills, 120–121
        problems with sensorimotor systems, 116–120
    performance areas addressed, 113–116
        problems with functional communication, 115
        problems with life tasks, 116
        problems with play and leisure, 115

Occupational therapy evaluation *(continued)*
        problems with school work and learning, 113–115
        problems with socialization, 115
        problems with work, 116
    in schools, 111–113
        common referral complaints, 112
Occupational therapy program implementation to remediate primary handicapping conditions associated with LD, 161–164
    speech-language therapy, 160–161
    service, levels of, 153–156
Organizational problems, 121
Organizational skills or study skills, problems with, 139
Otis-Lennon Mental Ability Test, 67

P

Parent interview form, 221–223
Parent's questions, answering, 210–212
    etiology discussion, 211
    prognosis discussion, 211–212
Peabody Picture Vocabulary Test—Revised (PPVT-R), 67
Peabody Individual Achievement Test—Revised (PIAT-R), 87–88
Perceptual-motor integration, definition of, 218
Performance areas addressed, 113–116
Play and leisure, problems with, 115
Postural control, poor, 118
Prenatal and perinatal history, risk factors for LD, 38
Preschool children, identifying learning disabilities in
    ADHD, 24–25
    behavior problems, 25–26
    diagnostic criteria, additional, 32–33
    discrepancy definition, 22–23
    discrepancy model for identification of, 27

Preschool children *(continued)*
    cognitive development, assessing, 27–28
        direct assessment, 30–31
        rating scales, 29–30
        specific skills, assessing, 28–29
        test performances, influences of, 31–32
    interest in, 19–20
    language problems, 23–24
    neurodevelopmental indicators, 26–27
Preschool Behavior Questionnaire, 29
Preschool-age children at risk for LD, identifying, 132–134
Primary (neurologically based) handicapping conditions, 4–7
    attention-deficit hyperactivity disorder (ADHD), 6–7
    learning disabilities, 5–6
    minimal brain damage (MDB), 7
Primary handicapping conditions
    definition of, 219
    diagnoses presentation, 206–207
    therapeutic recommendations presentation, 208–209
Professionals and families, role of in transition for adolescents with LD, 196–198
Psychological evaluation, differences with educational evaluation, 83–84
Psychological evaluation for LD
    history taking, 57–58
    testing, 59–81
        administration, 68–72
        interpretation, 73–81
        selection, 59–68
Psychotherapy for behavior problems, 188
Psychotropic medication for management of ADHD, use of, 175–179
Public Law 94–142, *See* Education for all Handicapped Children Act
Public Law 99–457, *See* Education for all Handicapped Children Act
Public Law 99–524, *See* Carl D. Perkins Vocational Education Act

Pupil Rating Scale—Revised: Screening for Learning Disabilities, 29

R

Rating scales, 29–30
Reading disability, 5
Reading disabilities, accommodations to circumvent LD, 165
Regression toward the mean
    concept of, 126–127
    definition of, 219
Remediate learning disabilities, educational approaches to, 156–160
    cognitive strategies instruction, 156–159
    direct instruction, 156–157
    social skills training, 160
Remediating primary handicapping conditions associated with LD, approaches to
    occupational therapy program implementation, 161–164
Revised Behavior Problem Checklist, 29
Rhode Island Profile of Early Learning Behavior, 29
Rule systems for language evaluations, 103–105

S

School, performance in, underlying factors in interference with, 116–121
    occupational therapy evaluation, 111–113
School work and learning, problems with, 113–115
School, behavior management system in, 186
Scores, standard, 125–126
Secondary handicapping conditions
    definition of, 219
    diagnoses presentation, 207–208
    therapeutic recommendations presentation, 209–210

SUBJECT INDEX 245

Secondary handicapping conditions, planning for treatment of
   behavior problems, managing, 182–188
   secondary emotional disturbance, managing, 188–190
Secondary program models for adolescent with LD, 192–193
Secondary school to college, transition, 198–199
Self-image, poor, 121
Semantics, definition of, 104
Sensorimotor systems, problems with, 116–120
Sensory and perceptual skills, poor, 117
Sensory input, poorly modulated responses to, 117–118, 119
Sensory integrative therapy, definition of, 219
Sensory Integration and Praxis Test (SIPT), 117
Sequencing, auditory, 108
Short-term memory assessment, 53
Slingerland Pre-Reading Screening Procedures—Revised, 30
Slow learner, 8
   definition, 219
Slow academic achievement, 6
Social skills training, 160
Socialization, problems with, 115
Soft neurological signs, 55–56
   definition, 219
Specific skills, assessing, 28–29
Speech-language therapy, 160–161
Standard Progressive Matrices, 67
Standard score, definition, 219–220
Standardized achievement and diagnostic tests, 86–89
   Kaufman Test of Educational Achievement (KTEA), 86–87
   Peabody Individual Achievement Test—Revised (PIAT-R), 87–88
   Woodcock-Johnson Psycho-Educational Battery—Revised (WJ-R), 88–89
Standardized norm-referenced tests, 85

Stanford-Binet Intelligence Scale, 28
Stanford-Binet test, 61–66
   Examiner's Handbook, 77
   subtest scatter and discrepancy among areas, 76–77
Stimulant medications for management of ADHD, use of, 175–179
Strategies Intervention Model (SIM) for adolescents, 193
Strengths and weaknesses in learning style, identifying, 134–135
Subtest patterns, common among children with LD, 77–81
Synkinesis, definition of, 220
Syntax, definition of, 103

T

Test of Early Language Development (TELD), 30
Test of Language Development Primary (TOLD), 30
Test performances of preschool children,
   assessing, 27–28
   influences of, 31–32
Tests, formal, used by occupational therapists when assessing LD, 114
Treatment of LD, planning for
   accommodations to circumvent LD, 164–167
   Education for all Handicapped Act and, 147–148
   Individualized Educational Plan
      components of, 149–150
      considerations for developing, 152–153
      developmental team, 148
      implementation of, 151–152
   Individualized Family Service Plan
      components of, 150–151
      developmental team, 149
      implementation of, 151–152
   remediate learning disabilities, educational approaches to, 156–160
      cognitive strategies

Treatment of LD *(continued)*
    instruction, 156–159
        direct instruction, 156–157
        social skills training, 160
    remediating primary handicapping conditions associated with LD, approaches to occupational therapy program implementation, 161–164
    speech-language therapy, 160–161
    service, levels of, 153–156
Tutorial model for adolescents, 192–193

V

Validity, definition of, 220
Verbal IQ-performance IQ (VIQ-PIQ), 129, 134
    discrepancy and subtest scatter, 73–75, 76
Verbal comprehension, auditory, 106
Vestibular system, definition of, 220
Visual perceptual/problem solving abilities, 44–46
Visual problem-solving abilities, 41

Visual/perceptual development, assessment
    block performance, 53

W

Weaknesses and strengths in learning style, identifying, 134–135
Wechsler Preschool and Primary Scale of Intelligence—Revised, 28
Wechsler Intelligence Scale for Children (WISC-R) test, 61–66, 78, 79
    VIQ-PIQ discrepancy and subtest scatter, 73–75
Wechsler Adult Intelligence Scale—Revised (WAIS-R), 65, 67
Woodcock-Johnson Psycho-Educational Battery — Revised (WJ-R), 66, 88–89
Word-attack skills, definition of, 220
Work Study Model for adolescents, 193–194
Work, problems with, 116
Written language disability, 5
    accommodations to circumvent LD, 166